Parkinson's Disease
A Guide for Patient and Family

Parkinson's Disease
A Guide for Patient and Family

Fifth Edition

Roger C. Duvoisin, M.D., F.A.C.P.
William Dow Lovett Professor and Chairman Emeritus (retired)
Department of Neurology
The University of Medicine and Dentistry of New Jersey
Robert Wood Johnson Medical School
New Brunswick, New Jersey

Jacob Sage, M.D.
Professor of Neurology
Director, Division of Movement Disorders
Department of Neurology
The University of Medicine and Dentistry of New Jersey
Robert Wood Johnson Medical School
New Brunswick, New Jersey

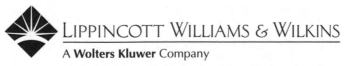

LIPPINCOTT WILLIAMS & WILKINS
A **Wolters Kluwer** Company
Philadelphia • Baltimore • New York • London
Buenos Aires • Hong Kong • Sydney • Tokyo

Acquisitions Editor: Anne M. Sydor
Developmental Editor: Stacey L. Baze
Production Editor: Jonathan Geffner
Manufacturing Manager: Colin Warnock
Cover Designer: Christine Jenny
Compositor: Lippincott Williams & Wilkins Desktop Division
Printer: R. R. Donnelley, Crawfordsville

Library of Congress Cataloging-in-Publication Data

Duvoisin, Roger C., 1927-
Parkinson's disease : a guide for patient and family / Roger C.
Duvoisin, Jacob Sage.—5th ed.
    p. cm.
Includes index.
ISBN 0-7817-2977-7
1. Parkinson's disease—Popular works. I. Sage, Jacob. II. Title
RC382 .D94 2001
616.8'33—dc21
    2001029689

Care has been taken to confirm the accuracy of the information presented and to describe generally accepted practices. However, the authors and publisher are not responsible for errors or omissions or for any consequences from application of the information in this book and make no warranty, expressed or implied, with respect to the currency, completeness, or accuracy of the contents of the publication. Application of this information in a particular situation remains the professional responsibility of the practitioner.

The authors and publisher have exerted every effort to ensure that drug selection and dosage set forth in this text are in accordance with current recommendations and practice at the time of publication. However, in view of ongoing research, changes in government regulations, and the constant flow of information relating to drug therapy and drug reactions, the reader is urged to check the package insert for each drug for any change in indications and dosage and for added warnings and precautions. This is particularly important when the recommended agent is a new or infrequently employed drug.

Some drugs and medical devices presented in this publication have Food and Drug Administration (FDA) clearance for limited use in restricted research settings. It is the responsibility of the health care provider to ascertain the FDA status of each drug or device planned for use in their clinical practice.

10 9 8 7 6 5 4 3 2 1

Contents

Preface

Our knowledge of parkinsonism has advanced in the four years since the Fourth Edition of *Parkinson's Disease: A Guide for Patient and Family* was published. To describe some of these advances, discuss some of the remaining controversies regarding treatment, and bring the book up-to-date required revising many of the chapters, rewriting the chapters on genetics and surgery, and adding a new chapter to address the question of whether or not levodopa affects disease progression. The result is a new edition, the fifth since the book was originally published in 1978.

The reader will find that genetics again has been placed "front and center" in the search for the causes of Parkinson's disease. Four years ago, before the first Parkinson gene mutation was found, we believed that one gene mutation might explain Parkinson's disease in most patients. At the time of writing, it is likely that many genes will play a role in the cause of Parkinson's disease, in the many symptoms and signs, and in the different rates of progression. Given the current state of the art of molecular biology and the human genome project, it is only a matter of time before many more gene mutations are found. The implications for all patients with parkinsonism and their families are great. Progress in finding a cause and a cure will be steady; however, it will take time and cooperation from patients and their families. We therefore felt it necessary to devote even more space to this new topic of genetics in parkinsonism in this Fifth Edition than we had in the previous edition.

At the time the First Edition was published, there were still many living patients with postencephalitic parkinsonism caused by the epidemic of "sleeping sickness" of the 1920s. Such people were depicted in Oliver Sacks's book *Awakenings*, which was later made into a motion picture of the same name. However, few, if any, "postencephalitics" survive today. Postencephalitic parkinsonism is now only a historical memory preserved in books and old journals. Yet due to its extraordinary nature, the enormous impact it has had on our understanding of parkinsonism, and the fear that it might some day return, we have retained a shortened account of this remarkable malady.

Although levodopa remains, after a quarter century, by far the most effective drug we have for the treatment of parkinsonism, drug treatment continues to evolve as new drugs and new formulations of older ones are introduced into medical practice. New formulations and ways of administering levodopa continue to develop. The use of the old anticholinergic drugs that were the chief form of treatment for parkinsonism prior to the advent of levodopa has since gradually declined. Today they are used only occasionally. Most have been forgotten and some are no longer available. New drugs designed to enhance or extend the effect of levodopa and to alter the disease process itself are under study. Some are likely to be in general use very soon.

The chapter on surgical treatment describes the resurgence of stereotaxic procedures. Stereotaxic brain surgery had largely disappeared after levodopa became generally available around 1970. In the past few years, however, it has staged a modest comeback. This has been due to new technology, an improved understanding of the deep grey matter of the brain (the "basal ganglia"), and the development of magnetic resonance imaging of the brain.

We have kept a focus on our basic knowledge of the clinical, biochemical, and pathological features of Parkinson's disease and on a historical perspective from our present situation. We maintain the belief that knowing the science of medicine and the way in which our knowledge has evolved over the years greatly adds to our understanding. It is a remarkable story of human achievement of interest in itself.

Jacob Sage
Roger C. Duvoisin

Parkinson's Disease
A Guide for Patient and Family

1

What Is Parkinsonism?

The word *parkinsonism* refers not to a particular disease but to a commonly recognized condition marked by a characteristic set of symptoms. Chief among these are trembling of the limbs, muscular stiffness, and slowness of bodily movement. To this triad may be added a tendency to stand in a stooped posture; to walk with short, shuffling steps; and to speak softly in a rapid, even tone.

The trembling usually affects the hands and feet but sometimes also the lips, tongue, jaw, abdomen, and chest. It tends to occur in the affected hand or foot when it is at rest and to disappear during a movement. For example, trembling ceases in the hand while it reaches out to pick up an object but reappears when the hand is returned to a position of rest. The trembling, or *tremor,* is thus a *resting tremor,* unlike tremors in other disorders.

The muscular stiffness is also of a particular kind. It is called a *plastic rigidity* because a doctor examining an affected person finds a constant, uniform resistance to passive manipulation of the limbs. The affected muscles seem unable to relax and are in a state of contraction even at rest.

The third element of the triad, the slowness of bodily movement, is called *bradykinesia* (from the Greek *brady,* meaning "slow," and *kinesis,* meaning "movement"). It is a very complex phenomenon comprising hesitancy in initiating a new movement or activity, slowness in its execution, and rapid fatiguing. The term *bradykinesia* also encompasses a lack of spontaneity and a decrease in the performance of automatic movements such as eye blinking, the swing of the arms while walking, expressive gestures of the hands while talking, facial expressive movements, and so on, of which we are usually unaware.

THE UNDERLYING DYSFUNCTION

This complex of symptoms that we call parkinsonism reflects the dysfunction of a particular region of the brain—in fact, of a particular system of nerve cells in a center, or nucleus, known as the *substantia nigra.* It is called the *substantia nigra* (from the Latin, meaning "black substance") because it is deeply pigmented; it may be readily noted by the naked eye in specimens of the human

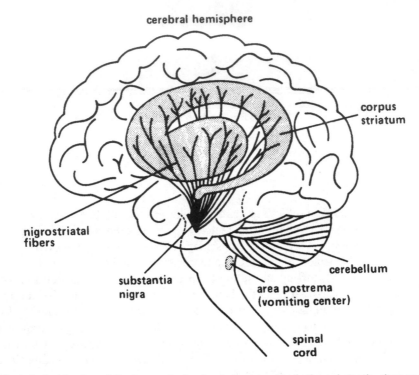

FIG. 1. Left-side view of the human brain showing schematically the substantia nigra and the corpus striatum (*shaded area*) lying deep within the cerebral hemisphere. For simplicity, only one side is shown. Nerve fibers extend upward from the substantia nigra and, dividing into many branches, carry dopamine to all regions of the corpus striatum.

brain. Under the microscope, pigment granules giving the substantia nigra its dark color can be seen densely packed within the nerve cells. This pigment seems to be chemically similar to the melanin pigment responsible for the color of our skin and eyes, and so it has been called *neuromelanin*. We believe that this pigment is related in some way to the fact that these nerve cells produce and store a specific chemical substance called *dopamine*. Similar pigment granules are also found in other nerve cells, mainly in cells that produce and store dopamine and the closely related substances adrenaline[1] and noradrenaline.

The nerve cells of the substantia nigra send long, thin fibers upward to connect with other nerve cells in the deep gray matter of the cerebral hemispheres known as the *corpus striatum* (from the Latin, "meaning striate body") (Fig. 1). Dopamine made in the cells of the substantia nigra travels up these fibers to the corpus striatum, where it acts as a chemical messenger transmitting signals to

---

[1]*Adrenaline* is the common name for this substance. Scientists refer to it as epinephrine. Adrenaline and epinephrine are one and the same.

the nerve cells of the striatum. When substantia nigra cells are injured or for some reason cannot produce or store dopamine, a deficiency of dopamine in the striatum results. If the deficiency is sufficiently severe, symptoms of parkinsonism begin to appear. Some neuroscientists have defined parkinsonism in chemical terms as a state of brain dopamine depletion.

A deficiency of brain dopamine can come about in various ways. The nerve cells of the substantia nigra may deteriorate for any of a variety of reasons. They may be injured by a tumor, a stroke, a chemical agent, or a virus infecting the brain (encephalitis). Brain dopamine deficiency can also be caused by certain drugs. A functionally comparable state can be caused by drugs that block the action of dopamine in the striatum. The dopamine then cannot deliver its chemical message, and the result is the same as when dopamine is deficient. Similarly, if the nerve cells of the striatum that normally receive the chemical messenger dopamine lose their ability to receive the message, the effect is the same as when dopamine is absent. This is believed to be the situation in certain disorders. Without going into further detail, it is clear that there are many possible causes of parkinsonism, some more important than others, and some very rare.

PARKINSON'S DISEASE

By far the most prevalent type of parkinsonism today is the condition first described by James Parkinson in 1817 in his "Essay on the Shaking Palsy." It is generally known as Parkinson's disease. It was the first type of parkinsonism to be recognized and remains the prototype against which other types are compared. It is sometimes called *idiopathic parkinsonism* or *paralysis agitans*. The term *idiopathic* means that the cause is unknown. Paralysis agitans is merely "shaking palsy" translated into Latin; it is the official name for the disease in the World Health Organization's International Statistical Classification of Diseases.

The cause of Parkinson's disease is not known. Pathologists classify it as a system degeneration of the brain because specific groups or systems of nerve cells appear to be the target of some morbid process. The disease process seems to select very precisely only certain nerve cell systems. It is clearly not a random thing. The location of the affected cells is such that their deterioration almost certainly cannot be due to poor circulation or to arteriosclerosis. Nor is there any sign of infection or inflammation. Under the microscope, however, pathologists can see an abnormal structure within the affected nerve cells. This structure was first described by Dr. Frederic Lewy in 1908 and so is known as the *Lewy body* (Fig. 2). These bodies are the hallmark of Parkinson's disease. They are not found in other forms of parkinsonism. The selective involvement of certain systems of nerve cells scattered through the brain and spinal cord suggests that an unknown toxin or a deficiency of some undiscovered nutrient may be responsible. Some think that there is merely a premature aging process that affects the cells of the substantia nigra. The truth is that the cause or causes are simply unknown.

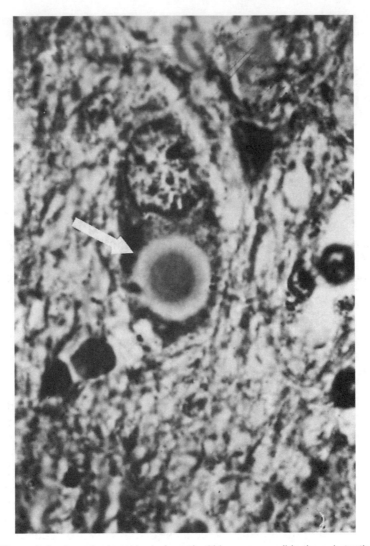

FIG. 2. Microscopic view of a Lewy body (*arrow*) within a nerve cell in the substantia nigra of Parkinson's disease patient. To the left is a large clump of neuromelanin granules. It is these granules that give the substantia nigra its black color.

The disease can affect people under the age of 40 years. The average age of onset, however, seems to be about 60 years. The beginning is usually so insidious and the progression so gradual that it can rarely be dated precisely. Usually, the first symptoms noted are, to quote James Parkinson, "a slight sense of weakness, with a proneness to trembling...in one of the hands and arms." These symptoms tend to increase very gradually over a period of many years. Indeed, progression is so gradual that little, if any, changes can be seen from one year to the next.

Parkinson's disease is believed to affect about 500,000 people in the United States, or approximately 1% of the population over 50 years of age. It occurs with a similar prevalence in other countries in which good epidemiologic studies have been done and appears in all races of mankind all over the world. It is difficult to make precise comparisons in different countries, however, because of differences in medical care systems and in statistical methods. Some statistical data are available in England and Wales dating back to the middle of the last century and from various hospitals and university clinics in the United States and several European countries at least as far back as the 1890s. These data suggest that the prevalence of the disease has not changed appreciably over the past century.

Occasionally, one encounters a husband and wife who both have the disease, but the incidence of conjugal parkinsonism is less than 2%, approximately what might be expected by chance alone. This is good evidence that the disease is not contagious. Moreover, since it may be presumed that husbands and wives have shared a similar diet and environment for many years before the usual onset of parkinsonism, this observation is also additional evidence that a dietary factor is not likely to be the cause of the disease.

Only a slight difference in the incidence of the disease in men versus women has been found. Moreover, studies of its incidence in different occupations or socioeconomic groups have not revealed any special concentration of cases. Parkinson's disease appears to be a democratic disease. The possibility that a virus may be involved in causing Parkinson's disease was once considered an attractive hypothesis. It has been suggested that an unconventional or incomplete virus causing a "slow" viral disease might be responsible. However, thus far no evidence for such a virus has been found.

The possibility that an environmental substance might be a cause of Parkinson's disease has seemed especially attractive in recent years, but despite extensive research no such substance has been found. The relative constancy of the prevalence of the disease over the past century argues against an industrial pollutant, herbicide, or insecticide as a causative agent.

It has long been recognized that some Parkinson's disease patients have similarly affected relatives. Many patients ask whether their disease is hereditary or runs in families. On casual inquiry, about 15% to 25% of patients report that they have an affected relative. On more careful study, however, at least half of patients for whom family information is available turn out to have affected relatives. Families in which cases have occurred over several generations are not uncommon. Thus, contrary to the prevailing opinion of only a few years ago, genetic factors are now thought to play an important role in Parkinson's disease. Recent research has increasingly focused on the genetics aspects of Parkinson's disease. These will be more fully described in Chapter 15.

In summary, the cause of Parkinson's disease remains unknown, but recent research suggests that the primary cause may be found in our genes.

DRUG-INDUCED PARKINSONISM

Another common cause of parkinsonism is the drug treatment of mental illness such as schizophrenia. There may be as many cases of drug-induced parkinsonism as there are cases of Parkinson's disease. However, they are almost entirely found among psychiatric patients. The powerful tranquilizing drugs used in treating mental illness block the actions of dopamine in the brain. The resulting disturbance of brain function is essentially the same as that caused by depletion of brain dopamine. The great value of these drugs is that they can tranquilize without causing sedation—that is, without making the patient feel drowsy, groggy, or sleepy. Introduced into medical practice during the mid-1950s, these drugs revolutionized the treatment of mental illness. They quickly displaced the padded cell, strait jackets, water therapy, and various coma therapies, such as insulin coma, that had previously been the main methods of treatment. However, these early drugs also cause a Parkinson-like state that closely mimics Parkinson's disease. Efforts to find an effective and safe major tranquilizer that does not cause parkinsonism have repeatedly met with disappointment. It appears that the tendency of these drugs to cause parkinsonism—blocking dopamine transmission in the brain—is fundamental to their effectiveness in treating mental illness. Some psychiatrists believe that producing a very mild degree of parkinsonism is necessary to obtain good results in their patients. It has been said, partly in jest but with more than a grain of truth, that treatment with the major tranquilizers represents a sort of "chemical strait jacket," more humane and more effective than the old physical methods. Two newer drugs in this category, clozapine (Clozaril, Novartis Pharmaceuticals Corporation, East Hanover, NJ, U.S.A.) and quetiapine (Seroquel, Zeneca Pharmaceuticals, Wilmington, DE, U.S.A.) do not produce parkinsonian symptoms and therefore can be used even in patients with Parkinson's disease. Unfortunately, quetiapine is not as effective as the other major tranquilizers, and clozapine may be toxic to the body's white blood cells, thus requiring vigilant monitoring with frequent blood tests.

The first of the major tranquilizers was the chlorpromazine, known by its proprietary names Thorazine (SmithKline Beecham, Philadelphia, PA, U.S.A.) in the United States and Largactil (Aventis Pharmaceuticals, Parsippany, NJ, U.S.A.) in Europe. Many derivatives of chlorpromazine have been made and are widely used as tranquilizers. These include trifluoperazine (Stelazine, SmithKline Beecham), fluphenazine (Prolixin, Bristol Myers Squibb, Princeton, NJ, U.S.A.), and thioridazine (Mellaril, Novartis Pharmaceuticals Corporation), to cite a few of those in more common use. One drug of this class, prochlorperazine (Compazine, SmithKline Beecham), is used mainly to combat nausea and vomiting. These drugs are known collectively as the phenothiazines. A closely related chemical family includes the drug haloperidol (Haldol, Ortho-McNeil, Raritan, NJ, U.S.A.). This is one of the most potent of the major tranquilizers and quickly induces parkinsonism.

One of the first tranquilizers found capable of causing parkinsonism was the drug reserpine, derived originally from the Indian snakeroot plant *Rauwolfia serpentina.* It was widely used for many years to treat high blood pressure. Although in large doses it can induce a state of parkinsonism, it very rarely does so in the small doses in which it is used to lower the blood pressure in hypertensive patients. Reserpine also causes a condition in animals that resembles parkinsonism, and it has consequently been used in experimental work to help find new treatments for human parkinsonism. Another drug used in treating hypertension, methyldopa (Aldomet, Merck & Co., Inc., West Point, PA, U.S.A.), produces a chemical parkinsonism, although this occurs very rarely. Both these drugs induce parkinsonism by causing a depletion of brain dopamine through chemical means. Metoclopramide (Reglan, A. H. Robins Company, Inc., Richmond, VA, U.S.A.), commonly prescribed for various stomach disorders in the United States, may also induce parkinsonism. It does so in the same way the major tranquilizers do; that is, by blocking the action of dopamine.

All these forms of drug-induced parkinsonism are reversible. The Parkinson-like state they cause gradually disappears when the patient stops taking the drug or if the dose is simply lowered. It may take several days or perhaps 1 to 2 weeks for the parkinsonism to subside. Rarely, it takes more than a month. We have never seen parkinsonism persisting indefinitely after treatment with any of the drugs we have discussed here. There is, however, one chemical agent, *N*-methylphenyl tetrahydropyridine (MPTP), that causes a permanent parkinsonism. It appeared briefly as a contaminant in illicit "street" drugs in 1982; only a handful of human patients with MPTP parkinsonism are known. MPTP has proved very useful in the laboratory to induce parkinsonism in animals.

POSTENCEPHALITIC PARKINSONISM

Encephalitis means literally "brain inflammation." In common medical usage, it refers to brain inflammation due to a virus infection. Parkinsonism occurring as a sequel to a viral infection of the brain is called postencephalitic, meaning that it came *after* the encephalitis. Only one kind of encephalitis is known to have resulted in chronic progressive parkinsonism. This was a rather unusual type of encephalitis that occurred primarily from 1916 to 1926 in small epidemics scattered throughout the world. A few sporadic cases were seen during the 1930s and the early 1940s. Only very rare cases have been seen since. The first cases were seen in central Europe in 1915 and 1916, and were studied and described by the Austrian neurologist Constantin von Economo. The condition was thus widely known as *von Economo's encephalitis.* Because it occurred chiefly in small epidemics, it was more generally called *epidemic encephalitis.* It was also called *encephalitis lethargica* because its first symptom was prolonged sleepiness.

In addition to sleepiness, the patients showed various types of strabismus, difficulty in swallowing, and bizarre changes in personality and behavior. Many patients, as many as 40% to 50%, died during the acute, or initial, phase of the illness. The survivors gradually recovered after 6 months or more, with various residual symptoms. Some remained severely crippled, with paralysis, tremors, severe muscle rigidity, marked mental changes, and many other difficulties. Many were thought to have fully recovered, but it was later realized that they too were left with subtle residual symptoms. They looked normal on examination, but their behavior was changed. They remained generally withdrawn and were unable to resume the pattern of their former lives and to return to school or work. They tired easily, had little initiative, and seemed generally passive. They were said to be "neurasthenic." Gradually, these survivors also began to show mani festations of parkinsonism. This delayed progressive phase of the illness was called chronic encephalitis, and later, postencephalitis. Because the patients had many symptoms similar to those of Parkinson's disease, they were said to have *postencephalitic parkinsonism.* This peculiar kind of parkinsonism developed in nearly all the survivors sooner or later, with the first symptoms appearing within 3 years in about 80% of them. Eventually, all the survivors had some degree of parkinsonism. They also had many other sequelae of their encephalitis that had never been seen in parkinsonism patients before. One of the most remarkable was the repeated occurrence of "visual spells," in which the head and eyes were turned up as if to look at the ceiling for hours at a time. These episodes were called *oculogyric crises.* Other unusual sequelae were compulsive tics and rituals that could be so severe as to render otherwise normal-appearing persons incapable of ordinary employment.

The first epidemics of encephalitis lethargica were observed in Europe several years before the great worldwide influenza pandemic of the winter of 1918 to 1919. There was, nevertheless, a common tendency to connect postencephalitic parkinsonism with the flu. No conclusive evidence was ever found that encephalitis lethargica was a consequence of the flu.

Repeated attempts were made to isolate an infectious virus from persons afflicted with this condition, but its cause was never found. Various viruses were recovered, notably the virus herpes simplex, which we now know is responsible for the ordinary cold sore. Initially, this virus was thought to be the probable cause, and a vaccine was prepared from it to treat cases of encephalitis lethargica. After many years of research and much effort, a great deal was learned about herpes simplex, but it seemed less and less likely to be the cause of encephalitis lethargica. Looking back at the efforts of the early "microbe hunters" to find the infectious agent of encephalitis lethargica, one can only admire how much was accomplished with tools that by present standards may only be called primitive. Clearly, the science of virology was not sufficiently advanced at the time to accomplish the task.

There were a great many patients with this type of parkinsonism during the 1920s and through the 1940s. In fact, postencephalitic parkinsonism was by far the most common cause of parkinsonism seen by physicians during those years. However, since 1950 new cases of postencephalitic parkinsonism have been very rare. The generation of individuals afflicted by encephalitis lethargica has now passed on, and this particular illness has disappeared.

No other type of encephalitis has been found to cause anything like the sequelae of encephalitis lethargica. Some symptoms reminiscent of Parkinson's disease are seen rarely during the acute or initial phase of various kinds of encephalitis, but these nearly always disappear during convalescence and never return. Very rarely, a few symptoms, such as tremor in one hand, may persist after recovery from some types of encephalitis (Japanese B encephalitis and central European tick–borne encephalitis), but these are mild and do not progress over the years, unlike the changes seen in survivors of encephalitis lethargica. Several types of viral encephalitis occur regularly in North America, usually in small, scattered epidemics. These include eastern equine encephalitis, western equine encephalitis, and St. Louis encephalitis. They occur during the summer or early fall and are caused by a virus transmitted to humans and horses by mosquito bite. The viruses responsible for more common illnesses such as measles, chickenpox, shingles (herpes zoster), and the common cold sore (herpes simplex) may also on rare occasion infect the brain and produce encephalitis.

Although all these viruses have been suspected at one time or another of being responsible for some cases of parkinsonism—even for parkinsonism developing many years later—there is no factual evidence to support these suspicions. And that is not for lack of trying. Many studies have been carried out in search of some association between parkinsonism and these viruses, so far with consistently negative results. An example is the long-term follow-up surveys of survivors of western equine encephalitis carried out over a period of many years by Dr. Knox Finley of California and the California Encephalitis Commission. Several cases of Parkinson's disease were found in approximately the number that would have been expected by chance, however.

Extensive studies of antibodies in the blood of Parkinson's disease patients were carried out by Dr. Teresita Elizan at the Mount Sinai Medical School in New York in the 1970s. The presence of antibodies to a specific virus indicates that the person in question has at some previous time been infected by that virus. More than 30 common viruses were studied, including several strains of flu virus. No evidence was found to implicate any of the viruses studied.

ARTERIOSCLEROTIC PARKINSONISM

Elderly persons who have recovered from several minor strokes may be left with some stiffness and slowness; a tendency to walk with short, shuffling steps; and some difficulty speaking clearly. If to these symptoms is added the gently stooped posture common among the elderly, there may be a resemblance to Parkinson's disease. Because the major problem in these patients is impairment of walking, they are said to have "lower-body parkinsonism." They are also said to have "arteriosclerotic parkinsonism."

This is a relatively rare cause of parkinsonism. Arteriosclerosis, or hardening of the arteries as it is popularly called, does not cause true Parkinson's disease. Usually, there is little difficulty distinguishing between the two conditions. However, sometimes the distinction may be difficult, and in an individual case even the experts may disagree. This is especially so in patients with a particular type of arteriosclerosis called *Binswanger's disease,* which primarily affects small cerebral arteries and causes progressive deterioration without overt strokes. Usually these patients have high blood pressure.

Of course, everyone more than 50 years of age has some degree of arteriosclerosis, and it is always possible to have Parkinson's disease plus some brain dysfunction caused by arteriosclerosis to complicate the situation. Arteriosclerotic changes are not uncommon in patients more than 70 years of age.

The differentiation of Parkinson's disease from arteriosclerotic parkinsonism is not just an academic exercise. It has practical value in judging the response to treatment. The symptoms of the latter do not respond to treatment as well as do those of true Parkinson's disease, and the elderly arteriosclerotic patients are more apt to experience side effects of drug treatment.

SYMPTOMATIC PARKINSONISM

A variety of diseases and intoxications can involve the substantia nigra, damage its nerve fibers on their long path to the corpus striatum, or injure the corpus striatum itself and thus cause some degree of parkinsonism. In such cases, the parkinsonism is considered a symptom of another disease. For example, brain tumors, if they happen to be in the right place, may rarely result in some parkinsonian symptoms. Similarly, head injuries, congenital malformations, and various infections, such as tuberculosis or syphilis, on rare occasions cause some degree of parkinsonism.

Certain types of poisoning tend to injure the corpus striatum selectively and may cause some symptoms resembling those of parkinsonism. The best-known disorders of this type are carbon monoxide poisoning and carbon disulfide and manganese intoxication. Victims of these intoxications may recover from prolonged coma with symptoms of diffuse brain damage, including some elements of parkinsonism. Parkinsonism has not resulted from chronic exposure to low levels of carbon monoxide. Manganese intoxication occurs chiefly in workers mining manganese ore. In recent years, it has been encountered in Taiwan and Chile but not in North America or western Europe. Manganese causes damage to the lungs as well as to the nervous system. The damage to the nervous system is extensive, and the symptoms include much more than parkinsonism.

The "punch drunk" state in oldtime boxers who have suffered repeated blows to the head also includes elements of parkinsonism. There is also a case on record of a man who suffered a bullet wound of the brain that destroyed the substantia nigra on one side. Symptoms similar to those of Parkinson's disease developed on the other side of the body and persisted for many years without further progression.

Rarely, parkinsonism occurs in adolescents or young adults (juvenile parkinsonism). Some of these cases represent true Parkinson's disease. Others are due to any number of rare hereditary disorders. One of these is a rare condition known as dopa-responsive dystonia, which usually presents in childhood with a disturbance of walking and twisting movements of the feet; parkinsonian symptoms develop later. This condition may be confused with juvenile-onset Parkinson's disease. The symptoms are completely controlled by very small doses of levodopa. Unusual cases of Huntington's disease appearing in adolescence may also mimic parkinsonism. Wilson's disease, a rare inborn error of copper metabolism, is another rare cause of juvenile parkinsonism.

PARKINSONISM PLUS

In many chronic progressive disorders of the nervous system, Parkinsonian symptoms may occur along with some other symptoms reflecting dysfunction of the cerebellum or other parts of the nervous system. These conditions are often called *parkinsonism plus,* the plus referring to symptoms that do not occur in true Parkinson's disease. These are clearly different diseases. The most common of these are progressive supranuclear palsy (PSP) and multiple system atrophy (MSA).

PSP was first described by Drs. Steele, Richardson, and Olszewski in Toronto, Canada, in 1965. In retrospect, the condition occurred many years before but had not been recognized. Considered a rarity at first, it is now diagnosed more frequently, and it is the most common form of parkinsonism plus. At first it masquerades as ordinary parkinsonism, but after several years additional symptoms appear. These include a very particular disturbance in eye movements that points to the correct diagnosis.

MSA comprises two conditions that often occur together: olivopontocerebellar atrophy (OPCA) and striatonigral degeneration (SND). These terms merely describe the pattern of atrophy or shrinkage that may be found on anatomic examination of the brain. In some cases of MSA, regulation of blood pressure, control of the urinary bladder, and sexual function are impaired. These patients are said to have Shy–Drager syndrome (SDS).

Collectively, MSA and PSP account for about 15% to 20% of all cases of parkinsonism seen in medical practice today. They are often very difficult to distinguish from Parkinson's disease in the initial several years of symptoms.

Progressive Supranuclear Palsy

Progressive supranuclear palsy (PSP) is the most common of the "Parkinson plus" syndromes. The initial clinical presentations may be like Parkinson's disease. For this reason, it is often first diagnosed as Parkinson's disease. The correct diagnosis is usually made several years after the first symptoms appear or not until after the patient dies and the brain is examined at autopsy. Patients with PSP complain of falls, gait disorder, visual problems, speech difficulties and swallowing abnormalities than do patients with typical Parkinson's disease.

Tremor is usually absent, and there may be a rigidity of the neck muscles that keep the head in extension. Patients have a wide-eyed, "astonished" stare that sometimes can be differentiated from the masked face of typical Parkinson's disease. The diagnostic criterion by which PSP may be recognized during life is the inability to look down voluntarily (hence, the name *supranuclear gaze palsy*). As the disease progresses, other eye movement abnormalities may occur. The treatment for PSP is generally the same as that for Parkinson's disease but tends to be less effective in the former disorder.

Multiple System Atrophy

Multiple system atrophy is the term now generally used to "lump" together what were formerly considered three separate conditions: OPCA, SND, and SDS. All forms of MSA may be characterized by parkinsonism in association with other, more atypical features. These can include an unsteadiness or imbalance and a disorganization of coordinated movements (ataxia or dysmetria) similar to that seen in normal people who have drunk too much alcohol. These problems with gait and balance appear earlier in the course of the disease than is generally seen with Parkinson's disease. In the SDS form of MSA, low blood pressure causing fainting and other signs of dysautonomia (urinary and sexual dysfunction) may precede or dwarf the signs of parkinsonism. Tremor tends to be less prominent than in Parkinson's disease, and perhaps most important of all, the response to levodopa is poor. Some patients may even worsen on levodopa.

ALZHEIMER'S DISEASE AND PARKINSONISM

Some patients with Alzheimer's disease may have parkinsonian symptoms. Occasionally, Parkinson's disease and Alzheimer's disease may occur together in the same individual. Such occurrences are thought to be purely coincidental. After all, both are relatively common disorders in those more than 65 years of age, and thus one could expect that some unfortunate individuals would simply by chance suffer both conditions. To complicate matters further, mental impairments similar to those of Alzheimer's disease develop in some patients with Parkinson's disease in which the cerebral cortex is also affected. These cases may be diagnosed and treated as Alzheimer's disease. It is extremely difficult in such cases to distinguish the two conditions. The correct diagnosis may only be made on postmortem examination.

Diffuse Lewy Body Disease

Sometimes a patient and family will be informed that a patient who has had Parkinson's disease for many years is developing diffuse Lewy body disease (DLBD). As the name implies, DLBD means that the disease is now spreading to many parts of the brain not usually involved with the pathologic processes of

Parkinson's disease. Although a definitive diagnosis of DLBD cannot be made except on postmortem examination of the brain for the presence and extent of Lewy bodies, the condition is often presumptively diagnosed in life by the presence of dementia, psychosis, and parkinsonism. The psychosis may consist of hallucinations, paranoid thoughts, and delusions. Dementia and psychosis suggest that the disease process has spread beyond the usual confines of more ordinary Parkinson's disease. As noted in the previous section, distinguishing DLBD from coexisting Alzheimer's and Parkinson's disease is not always straightforward.

Normal Pressure Hydrocephalus

Normal pressure hydrocephalus (NPH) is an uncommon syndrome that can resemble the other atypical parkinsonisms in that a disorder of gait is one of the prominent symptoms. Two additional classic features of NPH are urinary incontinence and dementia. It is caused by enlargement of the fluid-filled cavities of the brain, with subsequent compression of the centers that control gait, urination, and cognition. A brain magnetic resonance imaging (MRI) or computed tomography (CT) scan is often the first clue suggesting a diagnosis of NPH. It is important to distinguish NPH from the other parkinsonisms because it is potentially reversible with a surgical procedure that shunts fluid from the brain to another part of the body (usually the abdomen). It is also very important to be as certain as is humanly possible that NPH is the correct diagnosis before resorting to surgery, since shunting procedures, especially in elderly patients, are dangerous and can lead to major disability or even death.

Cortical–Basal Ganglionic Degeneration

Cortical–basal ganglionic degeneration (CBGD) is another rare form of parkinsonism in which a prominent feature is the marked asymmetry of symptoms and signs. It is important to remember that in most patients, classic Lewy body Parkinson's disease also starts on one side of the body but eventually becomes more symmetrical. For example, the resting tremor of Parkinson's disease usually starts in one hand and spreads to the other side. Even late in the course of Parkinson's disease, one side may be affected more than the other. In CBGD, this asymmetry is profound and continues throughout the illness. Furthermore, patients with CBGD may have other signs not usually seen in Parkinson's disease. These include a foreign feeling of involuntary positioning of the limb (alien limb phenomenon), loss of knowing what to do with the hand (forgetting the movements needed to brush one's teeth or comb one's hair; this is called *apraxia*), loss of sensations on the involved side, marked twisting of the limbs with the resultant posture becoming fixed and painful (dystonia), and extreme stiffness not often seen in the other forms of parkinsonism. Dementia and problems with gait and balance may occur. CBGD rarely occurs before 50 years of age and the course is relatively short. There is no effective treatment.

Benign Essential Tremor

Benign essential tremor (ET) must be mentioned here because some patients with presumed ET eventually develop Parkinson's disease. Patients with ET note that the tremor is of a different quality than those of Parkinson's disease. Essential tremor is worst on action, less severe on holding a posture, and rare at rest. The hands are usually affected and there is often involvement of the head and voice. The head tends to move in either a yes–yes or a no–no motions, and the voice has a vibratory quality. It is very likely that patients with essential tremor have several other family members with the same condition. It is thought to be a dominantly inherited condition in most patients. (Fifty percent of children of an affected parent are likely to inherit the condition.) Unlike the situation in Parkinson's disease, there is no slowness, stiffness, or significant imbalance. In those patients first considered to have ET and who eventually are diagnosed with Parkinson's disease, the course tends to be much milder and slower than usual. Presumably, these patients with an initial diagnosis of ET had Parkinson's disease from the beginning, but with a postural or action tremor rather than a rest tremor as the first sign. Hence, the difficulty in making the correct diagnosis until later, when some of the other signs of Parkinson's disease have appeared. (For another perspective, see the discussion of ET in Chapter 3.)

SUMMARY

Parkinson's disease has been known for nearly 180 years. Most authorities believe it is a specific disease. Although its cause is not yet known, it is believed that genetic factors play an important role. In addition, many disorders resemble Parkinson's disease to varying degrees. In some, the cause is known. There is also the remarkable fact that several groups of drugs can produce a condition that closely resembles Parkinson's disease but that disappears when the drugs are discontinued.

All these conditions resembling Parkinson's disease are called parkinsonism. Thus there is a postencephalitic parkinsonism, drug-induced parkinsonism, arteriosclerotic parkinsonism, and so on. Most of these forms of parkinsonism share one thing in common with Parkinson's disease: A particular set of nerve cells in a center called the *substantia nigra* are injured or impaired, with the result that the brain is depleted of a chemical substance known as dopamine.

2

The First Symptoms

So gradual and insidious is the onset of Parkinson's disease that patients can rarely pinpoint the precise date it began. At best, they remember when they first became aware of its presence. In many cases, the first signs of the disorder appear long before the patient suspects that anything is amiss. Sometimes one can find evidence that the disorder may have begun several or even many years before its symptoms are recognized. For example, on reviewing old home movies or videos, one can see that a patient failed to swing one arm while walking 5 or 6 years before tremor appeared in that arm. Old snapshots may show that the patient began to have a stooped posture many years before anything was suspected.

One of our patients had once consulted a speech therapist because of "mumbling" speech that made his work as a salesman difficult. Eight years later, he developed tremor in one hand and consulted a neurologist. The examination revealed tremor of the hand accompanied by rigidity of the arm as well as a soft, "mumbly" speech. It was then clear that the mumbly speech had, in fact, been the first manifestation of Parkinson's disease in that patient, but no one suspected the correct diagnosis until the tremor appeared. It is unlikely that even the most observant diagnostician could have found sufficient evidence to make the diagnosis when mumbly speech was the only problem.

Strangely, often the first sign of parkinsonism is noted not by the patient but by someone else. Usually, it is someone close to the patient—a spouse, relative, friend, or colleague at work—who notices some change. Perhaps there has been a subtle change in posture, stiffness of one leg when walking, or a new habit, such as holding one arm bent at the elbow and close to the body while walking. The patient usually denies that anything is the matter when asked about these things. A colleague may ask, "Is anything wrong with your leg? You seem to be limping." Or the patient's spouse repeatedly says: "Stand up straight. You're always bent over lately." Friends and family are often surprised that the patient seems unaware of these changes in posture or manner of walking or moving. They may prevail upon the patient to see a doctor. The interview in the doctor's office may go something like this:

Doctor: Well, what brings you in today?

Patient: Nothing, really.

Doctor: Nothing?

Patient: I feel perfectly well. There's nothing the matter with me.

The patient's spouse may then intervene to describe the cause of her concern: "Doctor, there's something wrong with his left leg when he walks."

So the doctor examines the way the patient walks. He may readily recognize the problem, but it often happens that the trouble is not apparent at the moment. Spouses often complain that the patient always looks much better in the doctor's office: "Doctor, if only you could see him when he is at home."

Most likely the doctor sees that something is indeed amiss, but the telltale signs of parkinsonism are usually not yet present at this stage of the disease, and the doctor probably cannot make the diagnosis. He may order a few tests: a blood count, the usual battery of blood chemistries, an electrocardiogram, an x-ray of the chest, and a routine analysis of the urine. This battery of tests constituting the usual checkup probably gives normal results. Parkinson's disease patients seem to be a pretty healthy lot, generally speaking. The experienced doctor probably wants to see the patient again in a month or two or if further problems arise. At this juncture, a little "tincture of time," to quote an old medical aphorism, is appropriate. If something really is going on, it should show itself more clearly in due course.

Eventually, the patient becomes aware that something is indeed wrong. There may be persistent tiredness, minor aches and pains, or a vague sense of malaise, of just not feeling well. The patient may feel a lack of energy or a sense of nervousness and irritability. Performance on the job may be declining for no apparent reason. The patient may notice that things once done with ease, without a thought, now require conscious effort. On seeing the patient again and listening to these vague complaints, the doctor can sense that there is a problem even though all the tests at the previous checkup were normal. He may try to reassure the patient that the tests were all normal. He may urge the patient to get some rest, perhaps take a vacation, and maintain a good diet. He may even prescribe a mild tranquilizer. If the patient seems depressed, the doctor may prescribe treatment with an antidepressant drug and suggest referral to a psychiatrist. Proper treatment of depression usually helps considerably, and the patient can carry on as usual for some time.

This phase of Parkinson's disease, in which vague, nonspecific symptoms develop, may continue for a long time. Some patients, understandably distressed by symptoms no one seems able to explain, tend to visit many doctors and clinics in search of an explanation, but the diagnosis is extremely difficult to establish at this point in the evolution of Parkinson's disease. The symptoms do not point to any specific condition. Overwork, lack of sleep, nervousness, depression, arthritis, poor dietary habits, and similar problems are more likely causes of such complaints.

Later, the patient may begin to experience more specific symptoms, such as soreness in one arm, a sense of weakness or "numbness" in one hand, stiffness in one leg, trouble in carrying out some movement, a change in the quality of the voice. There are almost as many initial symptoms as there are patients. Each individual experiences the disorder differently and interprets the experience in his or her own way. Although these more specific complaints indicate to the doctor that something is definitely wrong, there may still be no physical signs to suggest the nature of the problem. Even if a change in facial expression or a tendency to drag one foot slightly when walking or to favor one hand is noted, the doctor still cannot diagnose Parkinson's disease. A single finding is not enough to establish the diagnosis, and as yet no blood test—or any other kind of test for that matter—can establish the diagnosis.

The diagnosis can be made with certainty only when the three characteristic signs are present: *tremor, rigidity,* and *bradykinesia.* Tremor is usually the first to appear. Initially, it may be minimal. It may be noticed only when the patient is fatigued or under some stress. Some patients feel the tremor for many months before it is visible. If the writing hand is affected, it is common for the tremor to be noted in the patient's handwriting. Every letter tends to show evidence of a very fine tremor. Usually, the handwriting is also somewhat small, a phenomenon called *micrographia.* In addition, the patient's writing tends to get progressively smaller on the page or even within a paragraph. The doctor may thus ask for a sample of the patient's handwriting to look for these signs. Occasionally, tremor appears initially in a foot, and rarely in the lips, tongue, or jaw.

A small but significant percentage of patients have little or no tremor. Rigidity and bradykinesia may then be the first symptoms. The patient may experience only a sense of weakness of a hand or leg. There may be difficulty with fine tasks, such as buttoning up a shirt or tying shoelaces. Patients whose work or hobbies require some degree of manual dexterity may become aware of a loss of ability. In those who do not have tremor, the diagnosis is more difficult to establish and may not be made until relatively late in the course of illness.

As soon as one of the three characteristic signs is evident, the doctor recognizes that there is some disturbance in the nervous system and, especially if there is tremor, will suspect parkinsonism. Depending on the symptoms, the findings on examination, and the patient's age and general health, the diagnosis of Parkinson's disease may now be evident at a glance. However, often it is not so obvious at first, and many other possibilities cross the doctor's mind.

In many cases, the symptoms concentrate on one side of the body. The patient, for example, may complain of weakness of the left arm and leg, and the doctor may have noted some evidence of such weakness on examination. In appearance, the patient with such symptoms—walking with some loss of left arm swing and tending to shuffle with the left foot—somewhat resembles a person who has had a mild stroke.

Sometimes patients convey an erroneous impression that their symptoms came on suddenly. One patient, for example, said that he had first noted trouble with his right arm and leg a month previously and that he was now somewhat better. He believed that he had experienced a stroke. However, his wife described a more gradual and remote onset of his difficulties. It seems that the trouble with the arm and leg had been present for at least a year or more. On further questioning, it became clear that what the patient meant was that the trouble had become important enough for him to pay attention to it about a month previously and that he had not been fully aware of it before that time. It is quite understandable that a patient who recounts that sort of story to his doctor may be suspected of having had a stroke.

Whereas the sudden development of weakness or other symptoms reflecting troubles in the nervous system tends to suggest a stroke, a slow, gradual, progressive development of symptoms suggests the possibility of some progressive trouble in the nervous system, such as a slowly growing tumor. The doctor may have some difficulty in deciding which of these serious possibilities is most likely, especially in patients with no tremor. Even if there is tremor, however, the doctor will want to be sure it is not a stroke or a brain tumor mimicking Parkinson's disease—that it is indeed Parkinson's disease. He or she may order some neurologic tests or refer the patient to a neurologist for a consultation.

The popular image of the specialist as an expert who can make the diagnosis of exotic diseases after briefly glancing at the patient is a gross exaggeration. Of course that does happen on occasion—some conditions, though rare, are readily identified when first seen. Parkinson's disease, when fully developed, is easily recognized. The consultant's task is not merely to make the diagnosis or confirm the referring doctor's impressions but to make sure that what seems to be parkinsonism is not something else. There is no need for haste. Parkinson's disease is not an acute illness or life-threatening. There is ample time to allow the consultant to consider the matter as thoroughly as necessary.

The most important element in making a medical diagnosis is the patient's own account of the symptoms—the "history." The history is more important than all the tests modern laboratory technology has made possible. It is even more important than the physical examination itself. The consultant may ask numerous questions in order to gain an idea of the way in which the symptoms developed. Some questions may seem silly or vague, and patients sometimes answer facetiously or try to guess what is in the physician's mind and so give the answers they think the doctor wants to hear. Obviously, it is best to answer as directly and accurately as possible. After all, the consultant can make a more accurate diagnosis when given reliable and correct information with which to work.

The neurologic examination is a variety of the familiar physical examination one undergoes during an annual checkup or a preemployment physical. A complete neurologic examination can be a time-consuming affair; the routine examination commonly done by practicing neurologists may require 30 to 45 minutes or more, depending on the circumstances. A great deal depends on simple observation: By the time you have walked into the neurologist's office and said "hello," he has already learned a number of important things about you. During the formal examination conducted after completing the history, the neurologist examines the eyes, ears, mouth, tongue, throat, and neck. He inspects and palpates the muscles in all four limbs and tests the strength of the muscles as well as their tone. He uses the reflex hammer not only at the knee but at other places: at the elbow, ankle, and maybe the jaw. Every muscle has a reflex. The eye muscles are tested by studying how the eyeballs move when you follow a moving object with the eyes. Your ability to perceive various sensations—such as a pinprick, the touch of a twist of cotton, the vibration of a tuning fork, and others—is tested. The examination of sensory function is an important part of the neurologic examination and can reveal some extraordinary things about higher-level function of the nervous system. Posture (sitting and standing), the character of your walk, the manner in which you get out of a chair, and the way in which you put on your clothes at the end of the examination are all observed. Finally, the neurologist usually administers some tests of mental function. These are generally simple items, such as a brief test of memory, abstract reasoning, and the ability to do simple calculations. He may ask you to repeat some numbers, spell some words, do some simple subtractions and multiplications, and perhaps interpret some old proverbs. These may seem silly and embarrassing but bear with it. The neurologist is concerned not so much with whether you answer correctly but with how you handle the task. It is also important for him to have some basic idea of the quality of your mental response to the ordinary problems we all have to handle every day. Most neurologists also ask for a sample of your handwriting.

The consultant can usually make a diagnosis or at least give a general outline of the problem and the measures that may be needed to pinpoint the diagnosis after completing the history and the neurologic examination. He may say: "I believe you have Parkinson's disease, but I'd like to carry out certain tests to rule out some other possibilities." Your own doctor may already have ordered these tests, and the consultant may want to review them before reaching a conclusion.

The neurologic tests may include a computerized x-ray tomogram (called the CT scan), or a magnetic resonance imaging (MRI) scan, as well as some blood tests. These tests do not require admission to the hospital in ordinary circumstances and may be done in the hospital outpatient department or a private laboratory. The CT or MRI scan of the head is unnecessary but may serve as a screening procedure in some instances. The chances of detecting a significant abnormality are small, but the test is harmless, and a normal result is reassuring.

CT and MRI actually show the internal structure of the brain. The CT scan is a type of x-ray procedure, but instead of using photographic film to display the image, a series of images is constructed by a computer from a tremendous number of readings taken by an array of radiation detectors. The patient's head is placed between an x-ray tube and the detectors, both of which are mounted on a moving gantry so that they can rotate about the head. The detectors can make hundreds of readings in precisely controlled positions. From the readings, it is possible to calculate the intensity of the radiation at each of hundreds of points inside the head. A vast number of calculations must be done to determine the intensity at a sufficient number of points to produce an image. The calculations can be carried out within several minutes by a computer programmed for that purpose. The computer then displays the image on a television screen. A series of images are normally obtained, and these are usually photographed on instant black and white film for study.

MRI works on a different physical principle. The subject is placed within the field of a very large and powerful magnet that causes all water molecules to line up parallel to the magnetic force, just as iron filings do in the field of an ordinary toy magnet. In the presence of radio waves, the water molecules release electromagnetic energy that can be detected by an array of special sensors. Images can then be constructed by computer in the same way as in the CT scan. No x-ray radiation is involved in MRI.

CT and MRI scans are useful in studying patients suspected of having Parkinson's disease or related conditions. They have the advantage of being able to detect not only tumors but also the scars of old strokes and changes in the structure of the brain that are characteristic of various disorders that can mimic Parkinson's disease. Thus, for example, they are helpful in distinguishing arteriosclerotic parkinsonism or parkinsonism plus from Parkinson's disease.

These several diagnostic procedures are commonly used to evaluate patients with symptoms indicating some disorder in the brain. All the tests are usually normal in cases of Parkinson's disease. The consultant considers the results of these tests, the history of the patient's symptoms, and the findings of the examination of the patient, and then arrives at the best possible diagnosis. Sometimes additional blood tests may be needed. Rarely, a case of parkinsonism with no tremor but only a general slowness in all bodily movement resembles a case of hypothyroidism. A few simple blood tests to measure the blood level of thyroid hormone are helpful in this circumstance. Usually, the consultant can say, "I believe you have Parkinson's disease" and can advise the patient on treatment. However, occasionally even the consultant, with the benefit of all the tests described, cannot make a diagnosis with certainty. He or she may wish to reexamine the patient in a month or two. This is not an unreasonable request. The consultant may need time to think about the case. Moreover, the passage of time may allow the disease to reveal itself more clearly.

We have both encountered patients we had to follow for several months or even a year before the diagnosis of Parkinson's disease became clear. One of these patients was a middle-aged woman who for several years had complained of burning pains in her legs while walking. She was thought to have some circulatory disturbance in her legs and was treated with various drugs to improve the circulation, to no avail. She was then noticed to have a mild tremor of the hands. But there was no rigidity, bradykinesia, or other signs of parkinsonism. The tremor was not of the "resting" type, and so one could not say with certainty that she had Parkinson's disease. Two years later, there was slight but definite rigidity in the arms and the tremor had changed to a resting tremor. It was then clear that the pains in her legs and the burning sensations were manifestations of Parkinson's disease, and not of poor circulation. These symptoms disappeared on proper treatment of her parkinsonism.

Some physicians believe it best to reassure the patient with very early symptoms of Parkinson's disease that nothing is the matter. They fear that the very name *Parkinson's disease* will frighten and depress the patient, and so they try to reveal the diagnosis slowly or in stages. These physicians usually advise some responsible member of the family or the family doctor of the diagnosis. Sometimes the families join in this conspiracy of silence or insist on it themselves. They ask the physician not to reveal the diagnosis to the patient. "Mother doesn't know she has Parkinson's disease," a concerned daughter or son may say, "Please don't tell her. We don't want her to know."

In rare circumstances, there are good reasons for such silence, but in general it is ill advised. Invariably, patients have been hurt and angered by the attempted secrecy. We say "attempted" because in most instances the deception fails. It did, however, prevent the patients from getting answers to their questions. Since the diagnosis could not be admitted, it could not be openly discussed, and the patient could not learn what to expect in the future, what treatment could be given, what the effects of treatment might be, and so on. He or she knew well enough that something was the matter, so protestations from the family and the doctor that nothing was the matter gave little comfort. Sometimes the examining physician suspects the diagnosis of Parkinson's disease, but there are insufficient signs and symptoms to make a certain or even presumptive diagnosis. In these circumstances, we often tell patients that Parkinson's disease is a possibility but not a certainty or even a probability and that waiting and careful watching constitute the most prudent course. Usually, if the patient's early complaints are really those of Parkinson's disease, the diagnosis becomes clear in 6 months or a year.

Once the diagnosis of Parkinson's disease is established and other possibilities are excluded, the patient and doctor are ready to discuss the prognosis. Predicting the future is at best somewhat chancy, but some discussion about what the patient may expect, how his or her life is likely to be altered, what the treatment may be expected to accomplish, and so on, is in order. Precisely what the diagnosis means to a given individual depends greatly, of course, on the person and the circumstances. Some patients, perhaps thinking of a relative or neighbor who may have had Parkinson's disease, may fear the worst and imagine that they will rapidly become severely incapacitated. This is, of course, an exaggerated view. In fact, the symptoms in most cases can be kept under good control for many years. Other patients may have a falsely rosy view. They may recall hearing about a new cure for Parkinson's disease or may have read a glowing newspaper account of a new drug treatment and are confident the doctor can make the whole thing go away with a few pills or injections. This is the other extreme.

Clearly, it is important for the patient and the family to attain a realistic view of the nature of the disease and the general outlook. Patients should not hesitate to ask their doctor questions. To this end, both patient and family must allow the doctor to be as frank as possible.

Many patients spend much time and effort wondering about the origin of their disease. Often they ask if it could have been caused by undue stress at work or at home, an accident, or some great personal grief. Questions along this line are quite understandable. They reflect the patient's attempt to grasp in some familiar or comprehensible form just what is happening. It is difficult for many to accept that in this age of incredible technical and scientific accomplishment we do not yet know the exact cause of this one disease or how to cure it. It is best to come to terms with this and approach it with a positive attitude. The late Sidney Dorros put it extremely well in the title of his autobiographical account of his encounter with Parkinson's: "accommodation without surrender."

Parkinson's disease cannot yet be cured or prevented, nor do we presently have the means to slow its progression. However, successful treatment can control the symptoms well enough to allow most patients to lead active and independent lives for many years. Meanwhile, research continues on many fronts. Indeed, we are confident that current research will soon clarify the mechanism of the disease and, in the years ahead, lead us to more effective forms of treatment than are available today, to methods of slowing or even arresting the progress of the disease, and even to methods of cure and prevention.

3

The Classic Triad

TREMOR

Of the three major symptoms of Parkinson's disease—tremor, rigidity, and bradykinesia—the most obvious and familiar is tremor. It is usually the first symptom to come to the patient's attention, and most commonly brings the patient to a physician. The hand on one side is usually affected; sometimes one foot is involved. Typically, the tremor occurs when the affected hand or foot is at rest. The shaking is regular and rhythmic, with a frequency of five to six beats per second. A simple, small to-and-fro motion of the arm or leg may be all that is obvious. More often there is a complex movement, with slight turning of the forearm and a back-and-forth movement of the thumb and fingers reminiscent of a hand counting coins or of rolling a marble between the thumb and forefinger. For this reason, the tremor has been described as "pill-rolling" in quality.

The tremor disappears when the patient is asleep or resting quietly. Thus it may be present only intermittently, and its presence reflects the patient's state of mind. Nervousness, being "under stress," or even the alertness induced by concentrating on a mental task regularly enhances the tremor. The patient may sit home reading the newspaper quietly and have no tremor at all until a visitor arrives. It is this aspect of the tremor that patients find socially embarrassing, and many avoid company for this reason.

Patients may feel the tremor even when it is too fine to be noticeable. It may be felt as a quivering or vibrating sensation. Tremor of the musculature of the abdomen is felt as a vibration or something "quivering inside." Tremor of the diaphragm or of the chest muscles is sometimes felt as "palpitations," and the patient may erroneously fear that something is the matter with the heart and so consult a physician for that complaint. Since the tremor can be detected by electrocardiography, it may obscure the electrical record of the heartbeat, making it difficult at times to evaluate the heart properly. The electrocardiogram may have to be repeated on another occasion.

Tremor may involve the tongue, lips, and jaw, but rarely does it cause shaking of the head or affect the voice. Tremor may be confined to a very small part (e.g., one finger). Some patients report that their tremor began in the thumb or index finger!

A characteristic feature of tremor is its variability. It seems to come in bursts and then subsides. The tremor of one part need not be synchronous with that in another. In fact, tremor may appear in a hand for a few minutes and then quiet down, only to appear in the foot for a while. Most patients are able to stop the tremor by an effort of will. Many have learned various tricks to stop it. A slight movement or change of posture may arrest the tremor for a while; eventually, it reappears after some minutes or sometimes longer.

Tremor in one hand disappears while the patient is walking if he or she remembers to swing the arm. It reappears when the patient forgets and allows the arm to hang idly at the side, as if tremor were a substitute activity. Holding something in the hand can also stop the tremor. One patient always carries a small package in one hand when out walking. He found that merely holding the small weight prevents the tremor, which he is anxious to conceal. Many patients attempt to hide a trembling hand. They stuff the offending hand into a coat pocket, sit on it, or cover it with a newspaper or some object or even with the other, nontrembling hand. Embarrassment at having a tremor is very common among Parkinson's disease patients. In contrast, those with "essential tremor," which is usually more obvious and sometimes strikingly resembles the Parkinson tremor, do not seem to share this sense of embarrassment quite so often or so markedly. Why one type of tremor is embarrassing and the other not is unclear.

Patients have told us that they are ashamed to appear ill to their friends or family. Others fear that colleagues at work or their boss might notice the tremor and draw unfavorable conclusions. Unfortunately, there may well be justification for the fear of letting the boss, or clients, or customers see the tremor. Doctors, lawyers, accountants, and other professionals with a Parkinson tremor say that their patients or clients seem to lose confidence in them after noticing the tremor. A clothing salesman was fired with the explanation that his tremor would make a poor impression on customers! On the other hand, many patients fortunate enough to work in family-owned businesses or to have knowledgeable and helpful coworkers or employers have continued their work successfully for years despite their tremor. There is a need for better education of the public regarding Parkinson's disease.

In the very earliest phases of the disease, tremor sometimes occurs only at infrequent intervals, during periods of great nervous tension. For example, one patient first became aware of a tremor of the hand after an auto accident while trying to jot down the other driver's name, license number, and so on. The tremor subsided and did not reappear for several years! Understandably, the patient asked if the nervous strain of the accident might have caused Parkinson's disease in his case. It is not surprising that similar observations led nineteenth-century medical writers to consider whether fright or "nervous exhaustion" might not indeed be a causative factor in Parkinson's disease. Now that we know much more about the organic basis of the symptoms of Parkinson's disease, we recognize that nervous tension may indeed increase the tremor or bring it out when it is otherwise not present. In exceptional circumstances, it may even reveal the tremor a few months or years before it might otherwise have been noted.

Tremor occurs in many conditions. The most common one that is sometimes confused with Parkinson's disease is *benign essential tremor.* (See Chapter 1 for further details.) Generally, the tremor of this condition occurs when the arms are held outstretched for a moment or during a movement such as reaching for the handle of a teacup. In contrast, the tremor of Parkinson's disease occurs at rest. In other words, essential tremor is a "postural" or an "action" tremor. The tremor also tends to affect the head as well as the voice. The head shakes rhythmically up and down as if the patient were constantly nodding "yes" or from side to side in a "no" tremor. However, the distinction based on the relationship of tremor to movement or position is not always so clear-cut. Some Parkinson's disease patients have an action or a postural tremor for several years before a rest tremor develops as well. These patients for a time may be erroneously labeled as having essential tremor.

The major point of difference between these two conditions, however, is that neither rigidity nor bradykinesia occurs in essential tremor. Thus a physician examining a patient who presents with the complaint of tremor looks for other signs as well, especially for bradykinesia and rigidity. Patients with essential tremor tend to write large letters and to write quickly, whereas Parkinson's disease patients form small letters and write slowly. One can often suspect the diagnosis from a handwriting specimen alone!

RIGIDITY

Patients often complain of a feeling of stiffness, which is perhaps their subjective appreciation of rigidity. Strictly speaking, rigidity is not a symptom the patient feels, but an objective sign that can be appreciated only by another person during physical examination for evidence of resistance to passive motion. A physician takes the patient's arm and gently bends and straightens it a number of times while asking the patient to relax. The physician is looking for resistance to passive motion around the elbow joint. There may also be similar resistance to passive motion at other joints: the wrist, knee, ankle, spine, and so on. A persistent resistance to such passive movement with a plastic quality is what we mean by the term *rigidity.* It has a very characteristic feel and cannot be voluntarily imitated by the patient. It differs from the type of resistance to passive motion encountered in spasticity. There is often a regular, jerky quality to the resistance, as if a ratchet gear or cogged wheel in the joint was being manipulated. Physicians know this as "cogwheel rigidity."

One can also see on looking at "rigid" muscles that they are constantly tensed in a state of sustained contraction when they should be soft and relaxed when not in use. The tightness and firmness of rigid muscles can be felt with the fingers.

The patient may be aware of the muscular rigidity not only as a sense of stiffness but as a tired, aching feeling, persistent soreness, a pain, or a cramp. Thus rigidity of the muscles of the head and neck is often experienced as a headache. Usually, it is felt mainly in the back of the neck, shoulders, back of the head, and temples. Rigidity of the spinal muscles causes back pain (usually low back pain), which is aggravated by the tendency to stand leaning forward. Constantly leaning forward places the spinal muscles under a mechanical strain. Anyone who tries to stand leaning forward slightly in the posture common to many Parkinson's disease patients soon pain. Rigidity of the muscles of the calf and foot is manifested as painful cramps, not unlike the common charley horse provoked by athletic exercise.

Rigidity of the muscles of the chest and shoulder is sometimes felt as chest pain. When this occurs on the left side, the pain may be misinterpreted as the pain of heart disease known as "angina pectoris." One of our patients visited many heart specialists who conducted numerous tests and could find nothing wrong with his heart. When some tremor and rigidity eventually developed in his left hand, the diagnosis of Parkinson's disease could be made, and it became apparent that the chest pain was a symptom of this disease. After treatment with levodopa, the pain disappeared.

Aspirin and similar ordinary pain-relieving medications usually do not provide much help for the pain associated with sustained muscle contraction. Physical measures such as heat and massage are often helpful, at least temporarily. The back pain may be relieved by a hot bath, a back rub, or a heating pad applied to the muscles of the back. Massaging the muscles of the neck relieves headache, and kneading the calf muscle may relieve leg cramps. Proper treatment of the parkinsonism gives the best and most lasting relief. Improvement of the posture is also important in alleviating back pain. The pain often disappears immediately when the patient makes the effort to stand erect. A problem here is that the patient soon reverts to a stooped posture and again has back pain. Exercises to improve the posture are thus helpful but must be performed regularly to obtain good results.

BRADYKINESIA

Muscular rigidity slows movement. Some years ago many physicians believed that tremor and rigidity accounted for all the symptoms of Parkinson's disease. Rigidity may indeed impede movement. All movement requires the cooperation of opposing muscles, some relaxing while others contract and vice versa. The failure of an antagonist muscle to relax obviously limits a given movement. Consider a simple movement such as bending the arm (Fig. 3).

The biceps muscle causes the movement by contracting or shortening; it is the *agonist* in this case. The triceps muscle relaxes and allows itself to be stretched as the arm bends at the elbow, and is the *antagonist* muscle. To straighten the arm, the reverse occurs: The triceps contracts and the biceps relaxes. Failure of

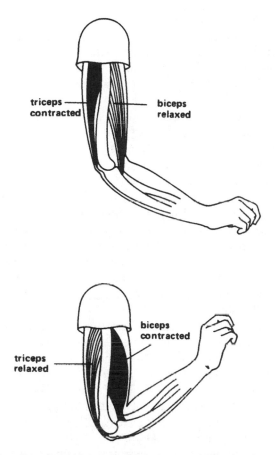

FIG. 3. Reciprocal action of agonist and antagonist muscles acting in opposing directions across a joint—in this case, the elbow joint.

the reciprocal action of these muscles is the essential feature of rigidity; that is, the triceps fails to relax on bending the arm, and the biceps fails to relax on attempting to straighten the arm. It is the failure of reciprocal relaxation of antagonist muscles that the physician feels as a resistance to passive manipulation of the patient's limbs. The rigidity impedes not only passive movement but active movement willed by the patient. It seems readily understandable that rigidity has been blamed for the slowness of movement (bradykinesia) in parkinsonism.

The reality is more complicated. If patients are observed carefully, it can be seen that slowness of movement may occur in the limbs with the least rigidity and that rapid movement can occur even with rigidity. Rare patients are observed who have bradykinesia but no rigidity at all. Thus, the two major symptoms do not parallel each other. Physicians once debated this subject at some length. The experience with stereotactic brain surgery finally convinced skeptics of the importance of bradykinesia. Many patients had excellent relief of tremor and rigidity, but in some cases relief of rigidity did not result in a corresponding reversal of bradykinesia. Rigidity was abolished, but good, rapid movement was not necessarily restored.

Physicians are sometimes surprised to see a patient who looks rigid but shows no signs of increased resistance to passive movement, no signs of true rigidity. This misleading appearance of rigidity is due to the complex phenomenon of bradykinesia, or more simply, akinesia (literally, "absence of movement"), a term that refers to both slowness and poverty of movement. When bradykinesia is minimal, it is barely noticeable and may pass for normalcy. Some people are normally slower in movement than others. Some are pokerfaced quite normally; others are very expressive. Since the range of normalcy is broad, a mildly brady-kinetic parkinsonian patient, especially if elderly, is apt to pass for normal. Those close to the patient, however, may have noticed a change. A man who was for-merly quick and vivacious and has become slow and deliberate may still be within the range of normal to a casual observer, but those who know him well are aware of an appreciable change.

Perhaps one of the most common manifestations of bradykinesia is the loss of automatic movements. These are movements that occur automatically, without out being conscious of them. They include the swing of the arms during walk-ing, eye blinking, swallowing of saliva, expressive movements of the face and hands, minor movements of postural adjustment, and so on.

A normal person who is sitting is not perfectly still. The eyes blink sponta-neously a number of times a minute. We are usually unaware of this or pay it lit-tle attention. The motor act occurs automatically without our consciously com-manding it. Similarly, we swallow our saliva several times a minute. We shift our weight from one side to the other, cross our legs, maybe even do little fidgety movements such as tapping the floor with our foot or drumming on the arm of a chair with our fingers. We turn our head and eyes from side to side to survey the scene around us. We clear our throats, nervously cough, rub our necks, scratch here or there. All these movements are done without significant conscious par-ticipation. A striking feature of the severely bradykinetic Parkinson patient is that these spontaneous motor acts are done much less frequently than normal. There is thus a poverty of spontaneous movement.

The reduced frequency of eye blink gives the face a staring expression. The eye blink functions as a sort of windshield wiper, removing bits of dust settling on the surface of the eyes. With reduced blinking the cleansing function is less effective and the eyes may become irritated. The eyelids become dry, reddened, and crusted, and the patient may experience a burning feeling in the eyes. Irri-gating the eyes with artificial tears or a suitable eyewash several times a day usu-ally alleviates this problem.

The diminished frequency of swallowing allows saliva to pool in the throat. When this is severe, saliva may spill forward in the mouth and pass through the lips, resulting in drooling. It was once thought that Parkinson's disease patients produced abnormal amounts of saliva, but measurements have shown that this is not so. In fact, they produce normal amounts but simply do not swallow it at the normal rate. Treatment with anti-Parkinson drugs improves the rate of swallowing and reduces the volume of saliva produced. The old anticholinergic drugs employed before levodopa was available dried up the saliva. Drooling was controlled but often at the expense of a feeling of dryness of the mouth.

Another class of automatic movements is associated with walking. Normally, one swings the arms while walking, each arm in synchrony with the opposite leg. Also, when turning, one "leads" with the head. The head and eyes turn first, followed by the shoulders, and later the trunk and legs. The bradykinetic patient fails to swing the arms or swings them to a lesser extent and fails to lead with the head on turns. Instead, the body turns in one piece.

Bradykinesia is also apparent in more voluntary movements. Here it is seen as a hesitation in initiating an action, then a slowness in the movement, and finally rapid fatigue, which is especially evident in repetitive movements. These features may occur in many kinds of motor acts. For example, if walking is affected, there is a delay in starting to walk. The feet seem glued to the floor. Finally, after several false starts, the severely affected patient walks slowly with shuffling steps. The steps become progressively shorter and then walking suddenly stops. Bradykinesia may be demonstrated in an affected hand by asking the patient to tap the knee alternately with the palm of the hand and the back of the hand. After a few false starts, the patient taps satisfactorily if somewhat more slowly than with the other hand. Then the tapping becomes slower, and finally it stops as the patient seems unable to turn his hand over fully.

Common problems caused by bradykinesia include difficulty getting up from a chair, getting out of a car, turning over in bed, and donning a coat or jacket. The activity begins all right but slows down and falters just before it is successfully completed. It is as if the energy required for the activity suddenly fails. Patients sometimes remark that they felt as if their batteries had run down. Other patients feel the bradykinesia as an external force restraining their movement. This is graphically shown in the self-portrait by an artist patient shown in Fig. 4. The patient has drawn ropes shackling her limbs to indicate her subjective experience of bradykinesia. Bradykinesia is also experienced as weakness or fatigue. It seems that the actions rendered difficult by bradykinesia can nonetheless be accomplished by an effort of will. This may seem fine to the person observing the patient, and one is tempted to encourage the patient by saying, "You see, you can do it all right." To the patient, though, it seems that something that should be done easily and without a thought requires effort and constant attention. One patient complained to me that getting out of a deep, upholstered chair required "a campaign of instruction to every muscle involved."

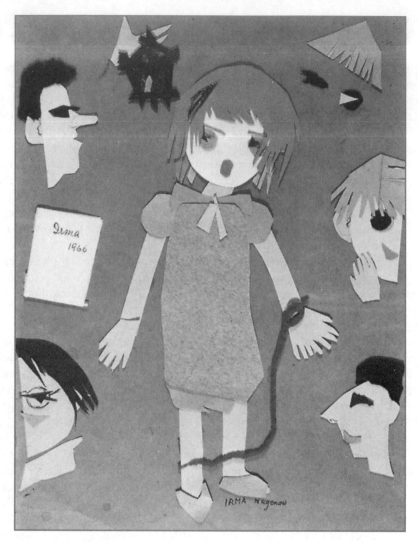

FIG. 4. Self-portrait of parkinsonism in collage by an artist-patient.

Another aspect of bradykinesia is difficulty in doing two things simultane-ously and in stopping one activity to start another. This is perhaps just another aspect of the need to concentrate on an ongoing activity to ensure its proper exe-cution. Ordinary activities such as dressing and eating therefore take longer than normal and appear to be done in a deliberate manner.

Bradykinesia varies considerably from moment to moment and in different circumstances. The patient can carry out an action or movement on one occasion but not on another. The variation is often quite striking in degree. The most strik-ing examples are known as *paradoxical kinesia*.

Every trace of parkinsonism seems to disappear for a brief period. The phenomenon is especially striking in severely affected patients. A chronic invalid who normally can barely walk with assistance suddenly walks down the hall normally, or a very ill patient requiring help to bathe and dress is found to have inexplicably gotten up early and dressed entirely alone. Understandably, such variability in performance strains the credulity of the patient's family or attendants. They are apt to refuse a later request for help in some minor task and say, "You did it this morning all by yourself, why can't you do it now?" Alas, the patient cannot do it now and cannot explain why. This is a common phenomenon in Parkinson's disease, but its mechanism is unknown.

The phenomenon itself has been interpreted as evidence that the parts of the nervous system that control and coordinate all motor activity are intact and that they can function normally if properly activated. The basic problem then must be in some defective regulation of those parts of the brain. Here we are at the core of the problem of parkinsonism, for bradykinesia is surely the most important symptom, even though it is not the most obvious one. It is also the most difficult to understand.

Many thoughtful physicians have tried to analyze bradykinesia. One of the great neurologists of the first quarter of this century, Dr. S. A. Kinnier-Wilson, thought of parkinsonian bradykinesia as a sort of "paralysis of the will." He came to this strangely metaphysical speculation because of the sense of effort and fatigue of which his patients complained. Such speculation, however interesting it might seem, does not help very much. What does *will* really mean? What connection is there between the material structure of the brain and a mental attitude or function such as will?

Other physicians saw patients' complaints that "everything becomes an effort" in another light. They argued that action was being blocked by some dysfunction in the brain. Far from the patients' lacking will power, they were in fact forced to rely on will power to overcome some central blocking or inhibiting effect. One eminent neurologist poetically observed that the patients were "condemned to voluntary movement." It has been noted that, in general, it is the automatic acts of daily life that are most affected by bradykinesia, and learned acts less so. Hence a severely bradykinetic patient may play the piano very well or execute a tap dance.

The late Professor C. David Marsden, director of the National Hospital for Nervous Diseases, Queen Square, London, England, has attributed the phenomenon to difficulty in organizing the series of motor "programs" required to carry out a motor "plan" in proper sequence. An apparently simple plan, such as a plan to walk down a hallway and pass through a doorway, requires a large number of changing programs. Typically, bradykinetic patients freeze at the point requiring more complex programs—at the doorway, where additional information regarding the location of the doorway, the number of steps required, and turning must be integrated into a smooth succession.

Professor David Brooks and his colleagues at the Hammersmith Hospital in London have studied the physiology of bradykinesia with an imaging method known as positron emission tomography (PET). They have shown that in normal subjects a small region of the cerebral cortex called the "supplementary motor area" becomes active shortly before a voluntary movement is carried out. Then the motor cortex becomes active during the movement. In Parkinson's disease patients, the supplementary motor area fails to activate until a dose of levodopa takes effect, restoring activation. Thus the dopamine system directly or indirectly regulates the ability of the cerebral cortex to initiate a movement. Perhaps this is where the "will" to move is located in the brain.

Every kind of activity may be affected by bradykinesia. It is hardly possible to describe all the specific manifestations of bradykinesia here. We can, however, take note of the basic elements of bradykinesia in whatever part of the body or type of activity is affected in a given patient at a given time.

4

A Plethora of Symptoms

There are so many symptoms of Parkinson's disease that it is difficult to mention them all in one volume. Many are uncommon or even rare, and few patients ever experience them. Some are fairly common but are more in the nature of nuisances than serious causes of discomfort or disability. Understanding their mechanism and significance renders them innocuous, although symptoms that seem minimal to one patient may be severe and distressing to another.

Many symptoms are only special instances of tremor, rigidity, or bradykinesia. Some of these were discussed in the preceding chapter. We can usually understand the mechanism of these symptoms quite readily, and understanding often reduces them to the level of a nuisance. Other symptoms are not so easily explained. We may simply have no real knowledge of their mechanism except that they are bona fide manifestations of Parkinson's disease.

ACHES AND PAINS

Parkinson's disease does not cause pain that requires a narcotic agent or powerful analgesic drug for relief. A variety of aches and pains do occur, however, and in extreme cases they can be quite distressing. Perhaps the most frequent symptom is an ache or soreness in an arm or leg that seems to be due to tremor and rigidity. The constant motion of tremor may represent a considerable amount of work done by the muscles of the affected limb, and it is understandable that the symptoms of muscle fatigue are occasionally experienced. This may not be the only explanation, however; patients may experience this symptom when tremor and rigidity are barely noticeable but not when the tremor is more prominent. A sense of aching soreness may precede the first appearance of tremor by a year or more and then disappear.

A persistent nagging muscle ache may accompany pronounced muscle rigidity. This too may be explained by the considerable work the involved muscles do in sustaining a constant state of contraction. Rigidity in neck muscles is experienced as headache, and in the foot or leg as a cramp. Usually, foot cramps occur during the night or on first arising in the morning. Foot cramps during walking are sometimes the initial symptom of parkinsonism. During the cramp, the muscles of the foot and calf of the leg are in spasm and cause the toes to bend in a clawlike position. The foot may also turn in at the ankle, and sometimes the first toe sticks up. This can be quite uncomfortable, especially inside a leather shoe. Rarely, a similar cramp may develop in the hand, usually provoked by tasks requiring fine control such as writing; it has been aptly termed *writer's cramp*. Rarely, a cramp in the neck muscles may cause wryneck, or *torticollis,* a sustained posturing of the head turned to one side. A similar bending of the head forward (*anterocollis*) may also occur, and, very rarely, a backward bending of the neck (*retrocollis*). These cramps and the resulting abnormal postures are known to neurologists as *dystonia* or *dystonic cramps.* There are, of course, many causes of dystonia, parkinsonism being only one.

Aching low-back pain is not uncommon in patients who tend to stand slightly stooped over. It is surprising how quickly the pain disappears when the patient stands truly erect or lies down; the pain may be worse in the sitting position because forward inclination of the back may be more marked in that position. Clearly, posture, as well as muscle rigidity, plays a role in this complaint. It is reminiscent of arthritis and is often erroneously ascribed to that disorder. However, the usual remedies for arthritis—aspirin, salicylates, ibuprofen, and simple analgesics—do not help, whereas they are quite useful to patients who really have symptoms referable to arthritis.

In addition to these various disagreeable sensations arising in muscles, some patients complain of a feeling of cold or, more often, warmth in some part of the body. It may be a hand, a foot, the throat, or one side of the body, or it may seem to be internal, as in the stomach or rectum. One of our patients experienced a feeling of coldness in his left hand for several years. The feeling came and went irregularly; it could be absent weeks at a time and then appear once or twice a day. Wearing a glove alleviated the feeling. Although the hand felt cold to him, its temperature felt completely normal on examination. There was no discernible difference in skin temperature between his two hands! Another patient complained of having cold feet at night for several years. He put on wool socks before going to bed every night, even during the summer. The symptom eventually disappeared.

A feeling of warmth is more common. Some patients experience a burning feeling in one hand or foot. An older woman who has had Parkinson's disease nearly 20 years complained frequently of a burning feeling in her throat and stomach. Extensive examinations failed repeatedly to reveal any cause. She had many x-ray studies of her esophagus and stomach, but there was no ulcer or the slightest hint of inflammation. There was, however, a connection between this symptom and her other symptoms. When for one reason or another her medications failed to take proper effect, her parkinsonism symptoms recurred, heralded by the burning feeling, which simulated heartburn. Tremor, rigidity, and trouble walking soon followed. Adjustment of the medication invariably resulted in disappearance of the burning feeling and improvement of all the other symptoms.

These strange temperature sensations were described more than 100 years ago as "thermal paresthesias." The medical word *paresthesia* means an "abnormal

sensation." The cause of these sensations is unknown except that they are gen-
uine, albeit uncommon, manifestations of Parkinson's disease. Narcotics do not
relieve them. There is no specific treatment for this symptom; generally, it
responds to treatment of the parkinsonian state as a whole. In one patient, spinal
anesthesia relieved the burning pain in the legs but blocks of the nerves in the
legs or of the nerve roots by epidural anesthesia had no effect. This suggests that
the pain arises in the spinal cord itself.

CHANGES IN POSTURE

Many patients with Parkinson's disease tend to stand in a mildly stooped posture. James Parkinson specifically mentioned this tendency in his introductory
definition of *shaking palsy*. He described it as a "propensity to bend the trunk
forwards" while standing and walking (Fig. 5). This posture does not develop in

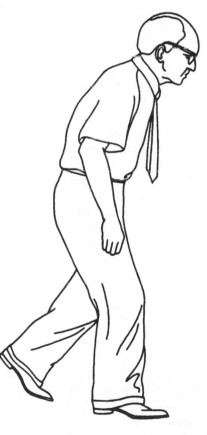

FIG. 5. This Parkinson's disease patient shows the typical "propensity to bend the trunk forwards" while walking, as described by James Parkinson.

all patients, and in many it is barely noticeable. On occasion, patients also tend to lean slightly to one side. This is especially noticeable in the sitting position.

Another common change in posture is a tendency to carry one arm bent at the elbow during standing or walking. If the patient makes an effort to swing the arm when walking, the posture disappears. It reappears as soon as the patient forgets to swing the arm. A less common postural change is a tendency to hold the foot turned in slightly. This is usually most evident in the sitting position with the legs at rest. Sometimes it can be noticed during walking.

Characteristically, patients are unaware of these changes in posture. They are sometimes quite surprised when they see evidence of their posture in a mirror or in a reflection in a window. This is not true of all patients, however. Some are acutely aware of the changes in their posture, and it is these patients who are of course in a better position to do something to minimize these postural abnormalities with exercise and sheer force of will.

PARKINSONIAN SPEECH

Many patients have no change in the character of their speech even after many years of Parkinson's disease, whereas in others the speech may be affected in a characteristic way. Rarely is this the initial symptom. The first change is usually a tendency to speak softly. The patient may have difficulty being understood on the telephone. Strangely, patients are often unaware that their speech is soft and are perplexed that others have difficulty hearing them. A loss of the normal volume of speech may not be troublesome to some patients, but others may consider it very important. It depends to some extent on the patient's life and work. A teacher, lawyer, actor, or someone who needs to speak or lecture notices the change in speech long before patients in other walks of life.

A patient who was a college professor complained that his speech was not sufficiently loud to be heard in a classroom. When he lectured, the students could not hear him, although his diction was fine. Since he simply could not project his voice anymore, he took speech-training exercises. This helped for a few years, but again the students complained that they could not hear his lectures. Finally, he obtained a throat microphone and a public address system. With electronic amplification of his voice, he was able to go on lecturing for many more years.

Another change in the character of speech is a tendency to talk in a steady, measured beat—in a careful, deliberate manner. Neurologists call this "monotone" speech. The natural song and cadence of speech seem to be lost. Some patients speak not only softly and in a monotone but also rapidly. The words are crowded together without the usual pauses between phrases, and the syllables are run together. When these three features appear together, the resulting *soft, monotone, rapid* speech is so characteristic that the doctor should immediately think of Parkinson's disease.

Some patients, however, speak slowly. Occasionally, the voice becomes lower in tone (i.e., hoarse), and sometimes higher in pitch. A rare phenomenon is a tendency to repeat a particular syllable in the middle of a word several times. It is similar to stammering yet different in character. The medical term for this is *palilalia.*

All these changes in speech are improved by effective drug therapy. They may also be helped by speech therapy. The softness of parkinsonian speech is due to a diminished movement of the chest. Normally, the chest acts as a bellows, forcing air through the larynx (the voice box) to produce the sound of speech, which is then modulated by the throat, mouth, tongue, and lips to form words (i.e., speech). Both rigidity of the chest muscles and bradykinesia affecting the whole action account for the diminished volume of speech. The rapid pace of monotone speech in parkinsonism is more difficult to explain, but essentially the same thing occurs in such other activities as walking, writing, and actions requiring repetitive movements. The tendency to diminished use of facial expressive movements and hand gestures during speech may further hinder the patient's ability to communicate.

SWALLOWING AND DROOLING

Akin to the problems of speech are changes in swallowing. The two, however, do not necessarily accompany one another. Swallowing is also a very complex act, although it is performed automatically. In Parkinson's disease, the complex sequential pattern of contraction and relaxation of the throat muscles necessary to propel food particles to the rear of the throat and into the esophagus may be slowed. The rate of swallowing is decreased. Consequently, eating may become slower and assume a deliberate quality. The patient must wait until the last morsel of food goes down before attempting to swallow the next. Foods seem to be held up at the top of the throat. Liquids and solids are equally difficult to swallow; soft foods seem to go down more readily. Attempts to hurry only make matters worse. Usually, it is necessary only to be patient and to eat slowly but steadily.

Slowing of the normal automatic act of swallowing one's saliva results in a pooling of saliva in the mouth and throat. When a large amount is allowed to accumulate, it may spill forward between the lips. The patient is then said to drool. Many patients feel that an excessive amount of saliva is flowing or being produced. However, careful measurements of salivary flow have shown that, in fact, these individuals form no more saliva than anyone else. Drooling occurs only because the patient fails to swallow at the normal rate. The drug treatment of parkinsonism usually results in both improved swallowing and a reduced production of saliva.

TROUBLE WALKING

Characteristic changes in the manner of walking occur in many cases of parkinsonism. The gait is generally less lively, the step is shorter, the foot is not raised to the usual height, and the automatic swing of the arm in time with the opposite leg is diminished or lost. Turns are negotiated slowly, sometimes with hesitation and with the body moving in one piece, whereas normally the head turns first, to be followed by the trunk and then the legs. When walking is more markedly involved, the toe may not be raised off the floor, and the patient consequently shuffles with one or both feet.

When walking is more severely impaired, several strange things occur. One may be called "freezing." The patient may be walking along very nicely when suddenly one foot seems to stick to the floor, firmly glued. After a few seconds, it is suddenly loose again. This annoying phenomenon may occur very rarely or frequently. A curious feature is that freezing tends to occur especially in doorways, while crossing the street, and on turns. When severe, it may precipitate a fall.

When the freezing phenomenon is prominent, the patient may have difficulty initiating the act of walking when first arising from a chair or getting out of bed. A number of very short steps, of an inch or so, are all that can be accomplished, and then suddenly the patient steps out with a normal step and walks normally across the room. The neurologist describes this pattern of rapid, short, shuffling ministeps as *festination.*

When long runs of festination appear, the patient may lean forward further and further as the steps become progressively faster and shorter until, after a dozen steps or so, the patient falls forward unless caught by someone or saved by a suitable obstacle. Some patients can use a cane effectively to stop the forward rush. The entire phenomenon is known as *propulsion.* When it occurs with backward stepping, it is called *retropulsion.* For example, the patient may make a few involuntary backward steps when backing out of a closet after hanging up a coat or when turning around a corner. For patients prone to retropulsion, wearing shoes with high heels may diminish or prevent the backward stepping.

The reasons for these disturbances of walking are not fully understood. Part of the problem appears to be an impairment of equilibrium. Walking has been described as a sort of controlled falling forward, with each step being a response to an impending fall. A common feature of patients with these problems is a diminished response to an impending fall. The normal responses to an impending fall are made too late, too slowly, and with movements too small. The normal responses—stepping, flinging the arms, and adjusting the position of the head and trunk—are normally done very rapidly and instinctively or automatically. Neurologists often test patients in the office for their response to a sudden gentle shove forward or backward. When suddenly pulled backward by the shoulders, the normal subject simply steps back, flings the arms forward, and bends the head and trunk forward. The parkinsonian patient with walking problems and poor equilibrium, on the other hand, fails to do these things and leans backward instead without stepping. If balance is especially poor, retropulsion may result (Fig. 6), or propulsion if the patient is pushed forward.

Usually, these walking disturbances respond fairly well to proper drug treatment. If necessary, physical therapy with emphasis on gait-training exercises

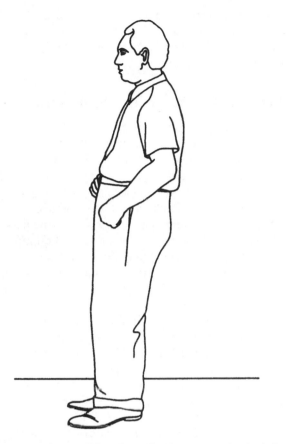

FIG. 6. In the phenomenon of retropulsion, the patient is unaware that he is leaning backward, thinking he is standing erect; he is about to step backward involuntarily.

may help. Shoes with rubber soles that do not slide easily on the floor may greatly increase the patient's difficulties.

CHANGES IN BOWEL HABITS

Slowness of movement seems to affect the bowels as well as the limbs and all bodily movements generally in parkinsonism. Constipation is a common and recurrent problem for many patients. Several factors may contribute to this. Many patients eat poorly, neglecting roughage and drinking little water. As a result, their stools become small, rough, and hard. This may make bowel movements painful and exacerbate any hemorrhoids that might be present. Constipation is usually only a nuisance, but careful attention to maintaining proper bowel habits fully rewards the little effort required. Rarely, severe constipation may respond only to enemas. Even more rarely, severe constipation is associated with enlargement of the large bowel or colon, called *megacolon*. This is due to failure of the nerve cells that regulate the constant activity of the muscles in the bowel. This can result in obstruction requiring a surgical procedure to correct the problem.

IRRITABLE BLADDERS (URINARY FREQUENCY)

The normal reflex mechanism for emptying the bladder may be overactive in Parkinson's disease patients. The reflex activates the detrusor muscle in the bladder wall that contracts to shrink the bladder and expel its content of urine. In Parkinson's disease, the reflex may be activated when the bladder is only partly filled. Urologists call this *detrusor hyperreflexia*. The patients experience a sense of urgency to empty the bladder as soon as possible. This urinary urgency is not uncommon. It is often more marked at night. Some patients say that they can hold their urine all day but need to go to the bathroom many times during the night. Various drugs with anticholinergic properties relieve this urgency. Urologists commonly prescribe oxybutynin chloride (Ditropan, Alza Pharmaceuticals, Palo Alto, CA, U.S.A.) or tolterodine (Detrol, Pharmacia and Upjohn Company, Bridgewater, NJ, U.S.A.).

Less frequently, some sluggishness of the bladder musculature may occur, so that urination may also be slowed. There may be difficulty in properly emptying the urinary bladder, and the patient may thus have to void again after a short time. Sometimes the patient allows the bladder to overfill, and then suddenly there is an overwhelming urgency to void right away. This is especially annoying at night, for it may necessitate getting up several times. Serious disturbance of bladder function is rare in Parkinson's disease. Should it occur, some other problem should be suspected, such as enlargement of the prostate gland in males or infection of the bladder or a "dropped" bladder in females.

SEXUAL DYSFUNCTION

Human sexual function is complex and intertwined with every aspect of life. It is a many-splendored thing, but it is also very intimate and personal and thus difficult to discuss with a stranger, even a physician. Perhaps this is why few patients complain of sexual dysfunction and why little is known of sexual problems in parkinsonism. Unfortunately, there have been few systematic studies of the problem.

The nervous system is involved in sexual activity at every level, from the highest to the lowest. Consequently, the nervous control of sexual function is susceptible to disruption at many points. At the highest level, psychological factors profoundly affect sexual behavior. For example, depression, anxiety, and frustration provoked by the very fact of being ill may sharply curtail libido. This is a common reason for sexual difficulties in many chronic disorders. Libido may be selectively impaired in parkinsonism by the disease process itself. Dopamine nerve cell systems in the brain seem to play some role in regulating libido. Patients have been described who have parkinsonism, loss of the sense of smell, and decreased libido. All three were improved by levodopa treatment. Although this combination of symptoms has not been systematically studied in Parkinson's disease patients, clinical experience suggests that it does occur in a small but significant number. The improvement of libido on levodopa treatment has been well documented (see Chapter 7). It may be partial, satisfactory, or sometimes excessive. Spouses have occasionally complained of exaggerated libido in patients when levodopa treatment is first undertaken.

Rarely, the nervous system is affected at a lower level, and the nerves directly controlling the sexual organs may be involved. In the male, the result is difficulty in maintaining an erection and delayed ejaculation. Comparable problems presumably may arise in female patients, but so far no evidence on the subject is available. These difficulties are often accompanied by other manifestations of disturbance in the nerves controlling vegetative functions, notably, loss of sweating in the legs and impaired control of blood pressure, the urinary bladder, and the bowel. This complex of symptoms develops mainly in some of the atypical forms of parkinsonism called *parkinsonism plus*. Indeed, impotence without loss of libido may be the initial symptom. Several of our patients experienced this phenomenon for several years before any sign of parkinsonism was evident. They had sought help at clinics specializing in the treatment of sexual dysfunction, to no avail. Unfortunately, this type of difficulty is not helped by levodopa. Urologists can help such patients with prosthetic devices and by various medications, the most effective being sildenafil (Viagra, Pfizer, Inc., New York, NY, U.S.A.).

Limitations of bodily movement imposed by rigidity and bradykinesia may cause problems simply by complicating the mechanical aspects of lovemaking. For example, slowness in turning over in bed may make it difficult for an affected male partner to assume a good position for foreplay or coitus. Rigidity and bradykinesia may hinder the pelvic movements necessary for coitus. Some accommodation to these difficulties can be made with forethought and the assistance of an understanding spouse, but they nevertheless deprive the patient and spouse of the natural spontaneity of normal sexual activity. Improvement of rigidity and bradykinesia with levodopa treatment restores normal sexual activity, chiefly by removing these mechanical impediments.

Many commonly used drugs—notably tranquilizers, antidepressants, muscle relaxants, and simple sedative and sleep medications—may impair sexual function. Drugs used in the treatment of hypertension and the drugs recently introduced for treating benign hypertrophy of the prostate gland in men can also impair sexual function. The anticholinergic anti-Parkinson drugs may also do this to some extent, at least in some patients. Usually, these drug effects result in delayed ejaculation and impairment of erection. Thus, if a sudden change in sexual function has occurred, it is well to consider whether it followed a change in drug treatment.

Many patients are afraid to discuss their sexual problems with their physicians (and vice versa). They tend to accept them as inevitable accompaniments of their condition or as a natural result of aging. But such may not be the case. Sexual dysfunction may be secondary to drug therapy or may result from an unrelated problem. Awareness of a problem may alert the physician to avoid certain drugs in planning treatment. We urge patients and their spouses to overcome their natural reticence and freely discuss sexual dysfunctions with their doctors. In recent years, especially with the development of sildenafil, specific medical treatments for male sexual dysfunction have proved helpful in many of our patients.

LOW BLOOD PRESSURE

In most patients, blood pressure is quite normal. Indeed, in our experience, hypertension occurs less frequently among Parkinson patients than among others of the same age. However, a small number of patients may have low blood pressure. Parkinson's disease affects the sympathetic nerves that regulate the heart and blood vessels and maintain blood pressure. If the involvement is sufficiently severe, low blood pressure may result, especially when the patient stands up. That is, the pressure may be normal when the patient is lying down or sitting but drops to a low level when the patient stands up. For that reason, it is referred to as *postural* or *orthostatic hypotension.*

It is very rare for Parkinson's disease patients to be aware of this low blood pressure, and it is not often recognized because blood pressure is usually measured in the sitting position only. However, if the blood pressure is sufficiently low, patients may experience symptoms of weakness, faintness, dizziness, or light-headedness on standing or walking, especially when first arising after sitting or lying for a time. The tendency to postural hypotension is exaggerated by drug treatment. It is usually easily controlled by various measures (see Chapter 7).

SWELLING OF THE FEET

Swelling of the feet sometimes occurs, usually appearing first and to a more marked degree on the side of the body where the first symptoms of parkinsonism had appeared years earlier. Usually, this occurs only in patients with a significant amount of bradykinesia. It seems to be due to diminished movement of the affected leg. The circulatory system relies on the effect of movement of the legs and contractions of the leg muscles to propel the blood in the veins upward toward the heart. If there is little motion, as in the patient who sits still all day, the veins in the legs become congested; some fluid then leaks out and accumulates in the tissues, chiefly in the feet and ankles.

This fluid accumulation is called *edema.* It usually diminishes overnight and increases during the day. If one presses down firmly on the skin of the ankle with the tip of a finger, it produces a small pit or depression that persists for some time. Physicians often search for this sign of edema when examining patients whose ankles seem swollen.

The swelling itself is usually mild in Parkinson patients and has no sinister significance. Sometimes patients think their legs are heavy and ascribe their difficulty in walking to the swelling. Of course, their swollen feet have nothing to do with their problems in walking. Occasionally, the swelling makes it difficult to put on tight shoes, but otherwise the problem is chiefly a matter of appearance; that is, it is "cosmetic." The edema usually subsides after proper treatment of the parkinsonism and as the patient becomes more mobile and moves the legs more vigorously. Sometimes additional measures are employed, such as use of a diuretic drug.

SEBORRHEA

Excessive discharge of the oily secretion of the sebaceous glands of the skin commonly occurs in Parkinson's disease. The forehead, the face at the sides of the nose, and the scalp are particularly affected. The forehead appears oily or greasy all the time, but more so in warm weather. The oily discharge may be irritating to the skin and cause redness, itching, and scaling. On the scalp, the scaling is recognized as dandruff. When the irritation is sufficiently annoying, it may be termed *seborrheic dermatitis*. This is a common skin disorder that occurs in many people who do not have Parkinson's disease or any other disorder of the nervous system. Dandruff alone is even more common. The various treatments (chiefly detergents and soothing lotions) commonly used for dandruff and seborrheic dermatitis may be used as effectively in Parkinson patients as in others.

EXCESSIVE SWEATING

Excessive sweating is another common manifestation of Parkinson's disease. It may affect one side of the body or even just one area, but it is usually generalized. The excessive sweating tends to occur in irregular bursts. It seems that the sweat glands are somehow poorly controlled and may respond to normal stimuli in an exaggerated manner. The tendency to excessive sweating is usually greatly reduced by treatment of parkinsonism. The mechanism is not understood.

HANDWRITING IN PARKINSONISM

Characteristic changes in handwriting that occur in Parkinson's disease may be of diagnostic value to the physician and a nuisance to the patient. The handwriting tends to get smaller. The letters are well formed but get progressively smaller as the patient continues to write; at the end, the letters may be so small that they are difficult to read. However, if one looks at the writing with a magnifying glass, the letters still seem well formed. This pattern may not be evident when the patient writes only a few words or a signature, but if samples of the sig-

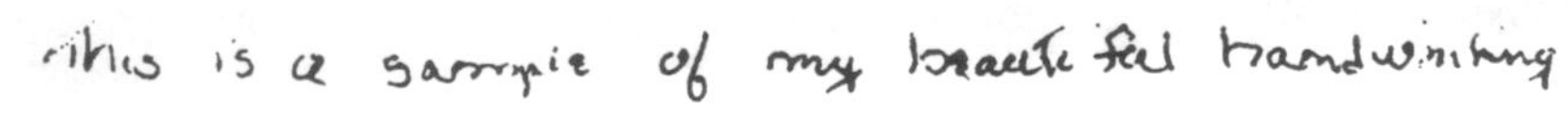

This is a sample of my beautiful handwriting

FIG. 7. Sample of handwriting showing micrographia. If one looks carefully with a magnifying glass, tremor is evident; look especially at the *f* in *beautiful.*

nature going back several years are examined, a change is often evident. The tendency to write small is called *micrographia.* In addition, if one looks closely, tremor may be evident in the writing in the form of very small squiggles in each letter (Fig. 7).

Effective drug treatment of parkinsonism produces marked changes in handwriting. It may become normal again, or it may be overcorrected so that now the patient writes in an unusually bold, large hand with extravagant flourishes. This is characteristic of the handwriting of patients with chorea and seems to parallel the appearance of drug-induced chorea (a subject discussed in Chapter 7).

VISUAL PROBLEMS

Occasionally, patients with longstanding Parkinson's disease complain of difficulty reading. They consult an ophthalmologist or an optometrist but are told their eyes are normal. They may need a new set of reading glasses, but aside from this, no ocular abnormality is found. Tests of visual acuity are normal. Sometimes patients are advised that the medication given to treat their parkinsonism may be the cause of their visual problem. This is, however, usually not the case. The oculists are simply unable to explain the patient's complaint.

One reason for difficulty reading is that the eyes do not move properly to scan a line of print. The eyes move in an irregular, jerky manner—slowing here, jumping ahead there—so the patient has to work hard to make out the sequence of letters and words. Then, having reached the end of the printed line, the patient has difficulty moving the eyes back to the left and down one line to find the beginning of the next line. Reading thus becomes a laborious task, and the patient soon tires of it. The problem is not in the eyesight itself. The optical properties of the eye have not changed. The problem is impaired coordination of the muscles that move the eyeballs from side to side and up and down. That this is indeed the problem can usually be ascertained with a little thought and careful analysis. There seems to be an analogy between the disturbances in walking and those in eye movement in parkinsonism. The eyes festinate, freeze, and travel slowly across the printed page while reading.

A rare phenomenon, ocular lateropulsion, may occur in which the gaze tends to drift involuntarily to one side, so that the patient has difficulty directing vision to the desired point. This seems analogous to the disturbance in equilibrium and walking called lateropulsion, in which the patient tends to veer to one side.

These disturbances in the coordination of the muscles that move the eyeballs are usually greatly benefited by levodopa therapy. However, they may not always be completely alleviated. Even so, marked impairment of eye movement is distinctly unusual in Parkinson's disease and, if unresponsive to treatment, suggests that a diagnostic reevaluation is in order. If there is obvious impairment of eye movement, the diagnosis may need revision or some other eye problem may have developed.

Very occasionally, a patient with Parkinson's disease may experience double vision. The patient sees two separate images of the world about him, each separate but overlapping the other, somewhat like the split image in a camera range finder when the lens is out of focus. This is due to the fact that both eyes are not looking at precisely the same point. This ocular phenomenon was common in the postencephalitic form of parkinsonism but may also occur, although rarely, in Parkinson's disease and other forms of parkinsonism. The problem is probably in the nerve cells that control the muscles moving the eyeballs. A curious feature is that the double vision tends to fluctuate. It may be present on some occasions, may be absent on others, and may vary during the day from minimal to marked. Spectacles with special prisms may correct the double vision. However, because of the variability of the phenomenon, some patients are helped by prisms, but others are not. The patient usually becomes tolerant of the double vision in time. The brain learns to ignore one of the images, and double vision is no longer experienced, even though it can be demonstrated by appropriate testing of the eyes.

There seems also to be a more subtle problem with vision in some patients that may be described as an "impairment of visual perception"; that is, there is some problem in the interpretation of the image cast on the retina by the lens system of the eye. The nature and significance of this dysfunction are not understood and constitute the subject of current research. The retina has a special group of nerve cells that contain dopamine. The possibility arises that the retinal cells may be depleted of dopamine in Parkinson's disease. Whether this depletion does in fact occur is still unknown, but it could explain some of the more subtle disturbances of vision that occur.

If one looks at a pattern of alternating light and dark bars or at a flashing light, changes in the electrical activity of the brain can be detected by electrodes on the back of the head over the part of the brain concerned with vision. These can be seen on the ordinary electroencephalogram (EEG), but computer analysis of the EEG is needed to sort out the visual effect from other electrical activities. The result is a characteristic pattern of activity called the *visual evoked potential* (VEP). The VEP may be abnormal in patients with Parkinson's disease. It is delayed and disorganized. The significance of this finding is uncertain, but it might be caused by depletion of retinal dopamine. It is interesting that the VEP returns toward normal after treatment with levodopa. Although many patients have an abnormal VEP, very few are aware of any impairment of vision, and they carry out ordinary activities of daily living without any evidence of defective vision or disturbance of visual perception.

The decreased frequency of eye blink in patients with Parkinson's disease may result in the annoying symptom of burning or itching of the eyes (conjunctivitis). The reason is that the normal "windshield wiper" function of the eyelids is not being carried out with the normal frequency. Thus dust particles, grit, smoke, and other irritants that are normally swept away with a blink are allowed to remain for an unduly long time. Consequently, the white of the eyes and the eyelids may become irritated. The eyes appear bloodshot, and crusts form on the edges of the lids. Irrigating the eyes with artificial tear solutions usually relieves these symptoms quite readily.

MOOD AND BEHAVIOR

Depression occurs at some time during the course of Parkinson's disease in about 50% of patients. Sometimes it is the first symptom, although this can only be determined in retrospect. Depression, of course, means a feeling of sadness, but it is important to remember that symptoms of depression also include loss of motivation, trouble falling asleep or early morning wakening, and decreased appetite with subsequent weight loss. Depression need not be constant; it can fluctuate from day to day or (particularly in advanced Parkinson's disease) even from hour to hour. It is easy to assume that this disorder of mood may be a reaction to the disease itself, and in small part this is true. We believe, however, that depression results from the biochemical deficiencies in the brain of chemicals related to dopamine (called *norepinephrine* and *serotonin*) that are responsible for mood regulation and are reduced in Parkinson's disease. The implication therefore is that most depression associated with Parkinson's disease is part and parcel of the disease itself and not simply a reaction to illness. The patient cannot help himself or herself and may need antidepressant medications to help his or her mood. Rarely, the depression may be so severe as to require electroconvulsive therapy (ECT). Sometimes the depression improves with anti-Parkinson therapy without the addition of specific antidepressants.

A small number of patients may get panic attacks, with palpitations, rapid breathing, sweating, and a feeling of impending doom. Generalized, low-level anxiety is more common than frank panic; both may require specific medications to reduce these symptoms.

HALLUCINATIONS AND PARANOID IDEAS

We have already mentioned in Chapter 1 that hallucinations (seeing people or things that are not there) can occur as part of diffuse Lewy body disease. In many instances, however, hallucinations begin as medications for Parkinson's disease are increased to combat progression of the motor symptoms. It seems likely that patients with Parkinson's disease are more likely to get hallucinations from the medications than are healthy people. Hallucinations usually are visual. The patient may see people, insects, or animals. Sometimes these people seen are strangers, but they may be the patient's children or friends. It is difficult or may be impossible for a spouse to convince the patient that no one else is in the room. The hallucinations may provoke paranoid ideas (a feeling that people are out to get you) in the sense that the patient feels threatened in some way; sometimes this elicits a violent response. Paranoid ideas may even extend to loved ones. A common paranoid idea is the belief that a spouse is unfaithful, stealing money from the patient, or trying to harm the patient physically. Treating these symptoms is imperative and will be discussed later.

DEMENTIA

Problems with memory, finding the right word, concentration, slowed mental responsiveness, mathematical ability, and other mental difficulties may occur in up the half of patients with Parkinson's disease. Often these symptoms are mild and not disabling. Late in the disease or in older patients, these problems may worsen and may lead to confusion and frank dementia. In such cases, patients need to stop working and may need specific help from family members. Dementia in Parkinson's disease can be severe (see Chapter 1 on diffuse Lewy body disease) but is usually milder than that seen in Alzheimer's disease. Confusion is frequently worsened by the anti-Parkinson's medications.

SLEEP DISTURBANCES

All human beings have a normal, if variable, cycle of sleeping and wakefulness during the 24-hour day. In patients with Parkinson's disease, this normal sleep–wake cycle is often disturbed, with resulting insomnia (inability to sleep restfully at night). Inability to fall asleep can occur but is less common than inability to stay asleep. Patients therefore wake up frequently during the night. There are two major ways to categorize sleep disturbances. Some patients have vivid dreams and nightmares and may thrash about and yell in their sleep. This often disturbs the partner more than the patient, but it may keep the patient awake as well as the spouse. Kicking and jerking of the limbs may also occur under these circumstances. Both the dreams and the nighttime movements are thought to be related to the effect of dopamine (usually from too much anti-Parkinson's medication). A second major difficulty leading to poor sleep is thought to be related to a lack of dopamine during the night (the opposite of too much anti-Parkinson's medications), which causes insomnia by the following mechanism. All of us wake a number of times during the night, during which time we change position in bed either by moving from side to side or simply moving the limbs into a more comfortable position. We easily resume deep sleep after each of these short awakenings. Parkinson's patients may awake but be unable to move well enough to make these small adjustments in position. The discomfort on being unable to move the limbs or turn over quickly and easily prevents them from going back to sleep rapidly and leads to insomnia. Other frequent causes of nighttime sleep problems include the need to urinate many times during the night and daytime cat napping. Excessive daytime sleepiness is usually due to reversing the normal sleep–wake cycle but is occasionally seen after doses of levodopa. In a few patients, pramipexole (Mirapex, Pharmacia and Upjohn Company) and ropinirole (Requip, SmithKline and Beecham Pharmaceuticals) have been reported to cause sudden onset of deep sleep during the day.

5

Principles of Treatment

The desire to take medicine is perhaps the greatest feature which distinguishes man from animals.

Sir William Osler

Over the long run, the patients who are the most successful in dealing with Parkinson's disease are those who enjoy a good working relationship with their physicians and families. The treatment of parkinsonism is necessarily more than the relief of specific symptoms. It is a cooperative undertaking, a joint enterprise of the patient, family, and doctor. Working together over the years, they seek not only to achieve the most satisfactory control of troublesome symptoms but also to make living with the disease successful as possible. Needless to say, the support and love of a concerned spouse and of the family as a whole make a great difference.

Ideally, it is best to continue with one physician, preferably the family doctor or an internist who can assume overall responsibility for medical care, and to rely on specialist consultants when the primary physician needs help for diagnosis, for specific advice about treatment, and for special problems. However, in the real world, the primary care physician, whether trained in family medicine or internal medicine, has had little training in neurology and is unlikely to be familiar with the complexities of Parkinson's disease and the drugs available for its treatment. It has been estimated that the average primary care physician sees fewer than three Parkinson patients a year—not enough to maintain familiarity with the condition. Thus it is best for the patient to visit a neurologist, not only to confirm the diagnosis at the outset and initiate treatment but also to follow the patient's progress over the years. We have found that follow-up visits every 3 to 6 months are adequate for most patients.

Many medical centers have groups of neurologists who specialize in the management of Parkinson's disease and related disorders. These are often called "movement disorder centers." Patients with unusual symptoms or those who have not responded well to the usual treatment programs may be well advised to visit such a center.

Continuity of medical care with regular visits and periodic checkup examinations is of great importance in a chronic disorder such as Parkinson's disease. It is a deplorable waste of time for patients to shop about from one doctor to another looking for a better or a new treatment without giving each new doctor sufficient time to become acquainted with and to learn the patient's individual reactions to the various treatments available. There are no secret treatments known only to one doctor or available only at a certain clinic or hospital.

There is no curative treatment for Parkinson's disease at present. Several years ago, the DATATOP (*D*eprenyl *a*nd *T*ocopherol *A*ntioxidant *T*herapy *o*f *P*arkinsonism) study suggested that treatment with the drug selegiline (Eldepryl, Somerset Pharmaceuticals, Inc., Tampa, FL, U.S.A.) (also known generically as deprenyl) might retard progression of the disease, at least in the early stages in newly diagnosed cases. Unfortunately, the preliminary finding was not confirmed on further study or in other, similar studies performed in Europe. However, the DATATOP study did conclusively show that vitamin E had no protective effect in the disease.

Although no curative or protective therapy is yet available, a number of drugs can substantially relieve the symptoms for long periods of time. The most effective and most commonly used is levodopa. First introduced in the 1960s, it remains to the present time the best and safest drug available for the treatment of parkinsonism. It is nearly always used in a formulation combining it with either carbidopa (Sinemet, DuPont Pharmaceuticals Company, Wilmington, DE, U.S.A.) or benserazide (Madopar, Roche Pharmaceuticals, Nutley, NJ, U.S.A.) to enhance its activity and prevent some of the side effects, especially nausea. It is commonly used as the initial treatment of Parkinson's disease. The symptoms can be so well controlled that progression of the underlying disease may be effectively masked for many years. Patients often forget what having parkinsonism is like. Unfortunately, if they discontinue treatment, the symptoms recur. Thus treatment must be continued indefinitely—essentially for the remainder of the patient's life or until someone discovers a better treatment or a cure. Additional drugs may be used to control specific symptoms not relieved by levodopa. Over the years, variations in the dosage and the daily schedule of medication or change to a different formulation (e.g., a slow-release preparation) may be needed to maintain the best results, but levodopa remains the mainstay of treatment in the great majority of patients.

Physical therapy or informal exercise is often helpful and sometimes necessary. There is no specific dietary or vitamin therapy, although attention to one's general health, and thus a proper diet, is as beneficial to Parkinson patients as to anyone else.

Brain surgery to relieve tremor and rigidity was largely abandoned after the introduction of levodopa 25 years ago, although it continued to be performed to a limited extent in a few centers. There is now renewed interest in brain surgery for patients with advanced disease or disabling symptoms, specifically in operations called *pallidotomy, pallidal stimulation,* and *subthalamic nucleus stimulation.* These procedures are useful in alleviating certain symptoms (see Chapter 11).

An important element of treatment is the interpretation of symptoms, as well as the advice and reassurance that an understanding and knowledgeable doctor can provide. It is essential to adjust one's life to the reality of the disease. All these things are important; in the final analysis, however, the cornerstone of effective treatment is the proper use of various drugs.

It is important that patients know a great deal about their medications. At the very minimum, they should know the names and dosages of each medication, and the time of day to take each one. They should understand why they are taking the medication and what results to expect. They should be aware of the major common side effects and how to deal with them. With such knowledge, patients can better cooperate with their doctor and so treatment can be more effective. However, treatment should be left to the physician. Self-treatment often leads to insuperable difficulties. Even patients who are themselves physicians should leave the treatment to another. An old aphorism has it that the doctor who treats himself has a fool for a patient and an incompetent for a physician. The wisdom of this familiar saying applies to all patients. Even if you do know something about the disease and its treatment, you cannot do a good job if you attempt to treat yourself. It is too difficult to judge objectively your own responses to treatment and to observe accurately your own symptoms. The days are gone, however, when the doctor simply tells the patient what to do and the patient just follows directions, with no questions asked. As we will see later in this book, there are many good approaches to the treatment of Parkinson's disease. Patients and families need to be informed about the pros and cons of various alternative approaches and should be able to participate with the doctor in making the decisions about treatment. A major reason to read this book is to gain sufficient knowledge that patients and families can make intelligent decisions together with their physicians.

Simply put, the drugs currently available for the treatment of parkinsonism act either by replenishing brain dopamine, mimicking the action of dopamine, or modifying the function of the brain in such a way as to compensate in some degree for the deficiency of brain dopamine. Dopamine is only one of many chemical messengers in the brain. Another messenger substance bears the chemical name *acetylcholine*. It is a very important substance. Indeed, there is much more acetylcholine in the brain than dopamine. It appears to be the chemical messenger for many nerve cell systems throughout the brain and is present in large amounts in the corpus striatum. Unlike dopamine, acetylcholine is not deficient in parkinsonism. On the contrary, there appears to be a reciprocal, seesaw relationship between these two messengers and their respective nerve cell systems. Dopamine is believed to act to restrain acetylcholine nerve cells. Dopamine deficiency in parkinsonism thus removes a restraining influence on acetylcholine nerve cells, and their unrestrained and consequently improperly regulated activity contributes to the various symptoms. Drugs that block or inhibit the action of acetylcholine tend to ameliorate the symptoms, whereas those that act by enhancing or imitating the action of acetylcholine cause an increase of parkinsonian symptoms. The opposite occurs with dopamine. Drugs that block the function of the dopamine nerve cells produce the disorder or make parkinsonism worse, whereas those that enhance these nerve cells relieve the symptoms.

Some of the drugs useful in the treatment of parkinsonism can be understood in terms of this seesaw relationship of dopamine and acetylcholine. On the one hand are the drugs that block the action of acetylcholine; these are the *anticholinergic drugs*. On the other hand are the drugs that enhance or imitate the action of dopamine; we will call these *dopaminergic* drugs. A very large number of drugs can block acetylcholine, and a few of these are recognized as anti-Parkinson drugs. Their overall efficacy is limited. On average, they can reduce the intensity of the symptoms of Parkinson's disease approximately 20% to 25%. They can completely abolish drug-induced parkinsonism. Several types of drugs can enhance the function of dopamine nerve cell systems. Perhaps one of the most familiar is amphetamine. However, amphetamine and its numerous cousins have very little effect in Parkinson's disease. Since amphetamines work indirectly by causing dopamine nerve cells to release dopamine, they might reasonably be expected to be ineffective when there is a deficiency of dopamine, and thus the poor effect of amphetamines in parkinsonism need not be surprising.

The most effective way of improving the function of the "sick" dopamine nerve cells is to replenish the depleted stores of dopamine. This is most easily accomplished by feeding patients the precursor substance L-dopa, which is converted in the brain to dopamine. (L-Dopa is the naturally occurring substance that is the active ingredient of the generic drug levodopa; for the sake of simplicity, the term *levodopa* will be used when referring here to this brain chemical; see Chapter 7.) Drugs that mimic the action of dopamine are also useful in treating parkinsonism. They offer the theoretical advantage of not having to be converted in the brain to the active substance; they act directly on the dopamine receptors in the corpus striatum, in effect imitating or substituting for dopamine. They are called *dopamine-receptor agonists*. They are less effective than levodopa but more effective than the anticholinergics.

One drug widely used in treating parkinsonism, amantadine (Symmetrel), is difficult to classify because we are not sure just how it works. It does not seem to have direct acetylcholine-blocking properties, although some evidence suggests that amantadine possesses indirect anticholinergic properties. It is thought by some researchers to act on the dopaminergic system, but this is unlikely in the doses used in humans. Its side effects and the symptoms of overdosage with amantadine are similar to those of the ordinary anticholinergic drugs. (See Chapter 6 for new use for this older drug.)

Selegiline, also known as deprenyl, was mentioned earlier as part of the DATATOP study. Although it does not have a protective effect on dopamine cells, it is useful in alleviating symptoms of Parkinson's disease. It works by blocking the "B" form of an enzyme called *monamine oxidase* (MAO-B). MAO-B helps break down brain dopamine. Selegiline slows the breakdown of brain dopamine and thereby increases the effectiveness of a patient's remaining store of dopamine as well as the effectiveness of brain dopamine derived from levodopa.

Other drugs that are useful in getting as much dopamine as possible to the area of the brain where it is needed are called catechol-O-methyl transferase (COMT) inhibitors. COMT breaks down levodopa in the blood. COMT inhibitors block the breakdown of levodopa in the blood so that more of it can get to the brain, where it is converted to dopamine. Two COMT inhibitors in general use are enta-capone (Comtan, Novartis Pharmaceuticals Corporation) and tolcapone (Tas-mar, Roche Pharmaceuticals). Unlike selegiline, which can be used alone, these drugs must be used in conjunction with levodopa; otherwise, they are ineffective.

A quarter century after it was introduced, levodopa remains the most effec-tive agent available for treating Parkinson's disease and most types of parkin-sonism; the exception to this is that it does not reverse parkinsonism induced by the major tranquilizing drugs. Sometimes we prefer to initiate treatment with levodopa; sometimes we prefer to initiate treatment with a dopamine-receptor agonist or selegiline. Less frequently, we start treatment with one of the anticholinergic drugs or with amantadine, reserving levodopa for more severe cases or for use later. The topic of initiating treatment is so important that we will discuss it in detail in a later chapter. There is general agreement among the experts that some form of treatment should be started when the patient has sufficient symptoms to affect lifestyle or employment. The treat-ing doctor must evaluate each case in the light of his or her personal experi-ence, and the doctor and the patient should jointly decide which way to go after discussing the pros and cons.

SIDE EFFECTS

Whichever drugs or combination of drugs is employed, certain general pat-terns of response may be expected. In advanced Parkinson's disease, much depends on the precise dosage and timing of the drugs taken. With proper care and diligence on the part of both patient and doctor, very good results can be achieved in most cases. The relief of symptoms can be striking. Usually, how-ever, some side effects must be accepted in exchange for the benefits. Naturally, some patients are more sensitive to the drugs than others. Some side effects are only mildly annoying; others can be quite distressing. Generally, the higher the dose, the greater are both the benefits and the side effects. The goal of treatment is to find the best possible compromise between the desired effects (i.e., relief of parkinsonism) and the undesired or side effects.

We should distinguish side effects from adverse effects. Side effects are nor-mal effects of a drug proportional to the dosage. Individuals vary considerably in responsiveness, and thus a given effect may occur at a low dose in some per-sons and at a high dose in others. In any single person, however, effects become greater as the dose increases. Some effects are desirable but only up to a point. After that they are undesired, or side, effects. For example, the reduction in salivary flow by anticholinergic drugs may be a desirable effect in a patient with excessive flow of saliva, but at a higher dose or in another patient, annoying dryness of the mouth may occur. This is then a side effect. Lowering the dose can reduce the effect to a desirable effect. In the same sense, drunkenness is a side effect of whiskey. One glass may produce a pleasant state of mind, but a higher dose produces the side effect of intoxication.

Side effects can be serious, even life-threatening, with whiskey as well as with the various anti-Parkinson drugs. Thus careful adjustments of dosage are necessary to obtain the balance between desired and undesired effects best suited to each patient. To strike the right balance is not always an easy task. The patient cannot do it. Another person who can see the patient objectively, preferably someone who knows something about the chemistry of the drug, its toxicity, its interaction with other drugs, and management of its side effects must do it. In short, the regulation as well as the prescribing of drugs should be left to the physician. In our experience, the patients who derive the best results from drug treatment are generally those who follow their prescribed regimen consistently.

Adverse effects are undesirable reactions that occur only in some patients. Usually, they are unrelated to dosage and are uncommon. They can be allergic reactions, such as those that may occur with any drug or food (e.g., an itchy, red rash may develop on the arms). Some adverse reactions are more serious, even life-threatening. When an adverse reaction occurs, the drug must be stopped. After the reaction subsides, treatment may be resumed with another drug, preferably one that is chemically unrelated.

A third type of undesired effect is sometimes caused by the interference of one drug in the action or metabolism of another. Some examples of drug interaction are given later.

RESPONSE OF SYMPTOMS

The symptoms of Parkinson's disease are not all equally responsive to drug treatment. Some symptoms respond quite readily, others less so, and some not at all. In fact, some symptoms may be exacerbated. For example, some anti-Parkinson drugs increase the tendency to constipation, common in Parkinson patients.

Patients often ask for a drug to control one symptom and another to ease another symptom, but the drugs do not work that way. It just is not possible to treat parkinsonism symptom by symptom. In general, the anti-Parkinson drugs act on the parkinsonian state as a whole, and they do not differ in their relative specificity for one or another symptom. It was once thought that some drugs were better for rigidity and others for tremor or akinesia. This line of thinking is reflected in the trade names of some drugs. For example, Akineton (Knoll Laboratories, Mount Olive, NJ, U.S.A.) (biperiden) implies an action on akinesia. Treatment based on such concepts led to complicated regimens that did not do any more good than simpler routines. Side effects are more frequent with multiple drug regimens, and it is generally easier to adjust the dosages of fewer rather than many drugs. If excessive side effects or adverse effects develop, it may be difficult to judge which of many drugs is responsible and which to stop or reduce. In short, it is better to use fewer drugs well than many not so well. It also is good practice, as well as common sense, to use drugs in the lowest doses that give a satisfactory result.

Generally, among the classic triad of symptoms, rigidity is the most responsive to drug treatment. Levodopa therapy usually abolishes it completely, often replacing it with hypotonia of the muscle. (That is, the disturbance of muscle tone we call rigidity is actually overcorrected!) The patient whose muscles are hypotonic looks "loose jointed" in bodily movements. The anticholinergic drugs can also alleviate rigidity, but rarely to the point of hypotonia.

Drug treatment reduces tremor greatly and often abolishes it. Of course, even if tremor is reduced by 80% or so, some tremor still remains and so the effect of treatment is not always fully appreciated. All the anti-Parkinson's drugs relieve tremor to some extent. Sedative drugs also alleviate tremor but to a lesser extent, and only at the expense of some drowsiness. Levodopa sometimes increases the tremor of Parkinson's disease at the outset of therapy, but with continued treatment it relieves the tremor more effectively than any other drug available today.

All the drugs reduce bradykinesia, or akinesia, and when mild or moderate, it is usually abolished completely. When severe, however, it may be only partially reduced. In patients with severe parkinsonism, akinesia is the most distressing persistent symptom. In these cases, rigidity is abolished and very little tremor is left, but significant akinesia may persist. Sometimes akinesia reappears briefly for a few minutes or so without tremor or rigidity.

Drug treatment can restore the automatic associated movements—eye blink, swallowing, swing of the arms during walking, expressive gestures, facial expressive movements, and so on—to normal or near normal. The amplitude of the voice and modulation of speech are improved. Disturbances of gait are also improved. The step becomes brisker, and the ability to walk slowly or rapidly and to turn around briskly can be restored. Shuffling, festination, and propulsion can be greatly diminished or abolished completely.

Feelings of numbness, weakness, aching or pulling pains, tightness, and so on, are relieved. The excessive sweating and oiliness of the skin are also diminished. Pooling of saliva and drooling are greatly ameliorated. Painful cramps and the rare heat sensations called thermal paresthesias tend to lessen but sometimes persist despite adequate treatment.

Because the disease continues to progress despite the best treatment possible, symptoms once well controlled may reemerge, or new symptoms may eventually develop. For example, a patient with only mild tremor and rigidity on one side when treatment was first begun may experience intermittent reappearance of the same tremor some years later; or a new symptom may develop, such as a tendency at times to drag one foot during walking. In such circumstances, patients often ask if the drug has lost its effect or if they themselves have become "resistant" to the drugs. Chances are it is merely a question of gradual progression of the disease, so that the duration of response to a given dose has decreased. As a result, tremor may reappear when the last dose begins to wear off. A change in the timing of the doses through the day or a change in medication (such as adding a dopamine agonist or COMT inhibitor if the patient is not already taking one of these drugs) will probably control the symptoms again. Sometimes a change in activity or diet may alter the metabolism of the drugs and render a previously effective dose less effective. In some patients, levodopa may be especially sensitive to changes in eating habits. Its absorption may be delayed by foods rich in protein. Thus, if there has been a sudden loss of benefit from an effective drug regimen, it is a good idea to check for recent changes in diet, lifestyle, or activity and also to check if the change coincides with the introduction of a new drug into the patient's regimen.

Whereas some patients require increases in the dosage over the years, others develop an increased sensitivity. Usually, the dosage of levodopa required, once established, remains about the same for years: After many years, it may be useful to modify the schedule of doses through the day. Somewhat smaller doses taken at shorter intervals may then prove helpful, or a change to the slow-release formulation or the addition of another drug (dopamine agonist, COMT inhibitor, selegiline, and so on).

Rarely, the drugs produce results opposite to those expected. They may relieve some symptoms at one dose and increase others at a higher dose. This is called a "paradoxical" effect. One of our patients, when first seen, was troubled chiefly by a slowness of movement and stiffness in his legs while walking. Treatment with levodopa at the modest dose improved these symptoms to a moderate degree. However, when the dose was increased further, he failed to improve. In fact, his wife reported that at a higher dose he was actually slower and stiffer. When the patient discontinued his medication for several days for a religious fast, he reported that he actually felt better. He then remained off his medication completely for several more days. Although he felt better at first, he gradually became worse again and all his original symptoms returned. He then resumed taking levodopa and found that he felt best at an intermediate dose. Puzzled by this observation, we admitted him to the hospital to study his reaction to levodopa more objectively. He was treated with a very small dose for several days, then with a full dose for several days. He was examined hourly during the day, and blood samples were taken to measure the amount of the drug. When the results were in, it was clear that he did indeed have a striking paradoxical response to levodopa treatment. The higher the dose he took and the higher the blood level, the greater were his symptoms: He was slower and walked more stiffly. When he set out to walk, his feet seemed to hesitate as if his shoes were momentarily stuck to the floor. This curious phenomenon has been called *start hesitation* and has occasionally been observed as a paradoxical effect in patients on higher doses.

Thus, if a new symptom appears after an increase in the dose, the possibility of a paradoxical response should be considered. In such circumstances, there may be a narrow range over which the dosage is optimal. Going above or below that range makes matters worse! Finding the optimal dose may require considerable patience and care in making dosage adjustments. It requires close cooperation of patient and doctor.

DRUG HOLIDAYS

It was first noted some years ago during the initial trials of levodopa that when therapy was withdrawn for 1 week or more and then resumed, it was more effective for a time. This observation led to the widespread use of "drug holidays" in the hope of restoring responsiveness to levodopa. However, with further experience, enthusiasm for the drug holiday declined. It proved useful only in the rare instances when patients had severe involuntary movements and mental disturbances. It may be a difficult, unpleasant, and even dangerous experience for the patient, and should be done only by a physician experienced in its use, preferably in the hospital.

6

Anticholinergic Drugs

For a century before the advent of levodopa, anticholinergic drugs were the only treatment available for parkinsonism. They have been largely supplanted by levodopa and other drugs. We rarely use them in our own practice. However, they may still be helpful occasionally in patients to supplement the effects of levodopa or in the rare patients who cannot tolerate levodopa. It is also important to be aware that the anticholinergic properties of drugs given for some other reason (e.g., antihistamines taken as a cold remedy) will have some effect on Parkinson's disease symptoms. Therefore, we should briefly review this class of drugs.

The first anticholinergic drugs were derived from plants. Just how they came to be used in treating parkinsonism is unclear. The first definite mention of their use for this purpose seems to be a comment in a doctoral thesis dated 1869 by a medical student in Paris, France, that Professor Charcot was then administering some hyoscine to patients with Parkinson's disease. Hyoscine, also called *scopolamine*, is the active ingredient of the plant *Datura stramonium*, known popularly as jimsonweed or thorn apple. Wine extracts of the plant had been used for centuries as tincture of stramonium in the treatment of stomach cramps and abdominal colic. Closely related botanical preparations are the alcoholic extract, or tincture, of the plant *Hyoscyamus niger* (black henbane) and the extract of *Atropa belladonna* (deadly nightshade). The active principles are named *hyoscyamine* and *atropine*, respectively. The plants are members of the potato family, called Solanaceae in botanical terminology. The extracts are alkaline and bitter-tasting; hence, they are termed *solanaceous alkaloids*.

Tincture of belladonna and its active ingredients (or principles), atropine and hyoscine (scopolamine), are still used for some purposes in medical practice. They act on the vagus nerve, which controls the stomach, intestine, bladder, and heart. The vagus nerve transmits its influence to the various organs through the action of a chemical intermediary, or messenger. The messenger is a simple chemical substance called *acetylcholine*. The solanaceous alkaloids work by blocking the action of acetylcholine and thus are classed as *anticholinergic drugs*.

For some unknown reason, patients with postencephalitic parkinsonism tolerated much larger doses of anticholinergic drugs than can normal people or even patients with Parkinson's disease. The postencephalitic cases were also quite numerous during the 1920s and 1930s. Thus particular attention was directed to their treatment. Various treatment regimens with these alkaloids were developed, such as Roemer's high-dosage atropine treatment, in which doses that today would be considered fantastic were routinely employed.

The high dosages of the drugs used produced side effects, including mental confusion, mild incoordination, slurred speech, and forgetfulness, which collectively were known as the "belladonna jag." Similar symptoms of anticholinergic intoxication may occur in Parkinson's disease patients with much smaller doses. Other side effects included blurred vision, dry mouth, inability to sweat, and constipation.

SYNTHETIC ANTICHOLINERGIC DRUGS

Once the chemical structure of acetylcholine was known, chemists could synthesize new chemical compounds in the laboratory to imitate or block its action. Thus synthetic anticholinergic drugs were developed in the hope that they would be more effective. One of the first of these drugs, trihexyphenidyl (Artane, Lederle Laboratories, Pearl River, NY, U.S.A.), was introduced as an anti-Parkinson drug about 1950. It appeared to have fewer side effects than the older potato plant drugs and to be equally effective. It was rapidly followed by three other closely related drugs: procyclidine (Kemadrin, Glaxo Wellcome, Schönbühl, Germany), cycrimine, and biperiden (Akineton). Of these, only trihexyphenidyl and biperiden are still available. Trihexyphenidyl is also marketed under different names.

For most of the 20 years from 1950 to 1970 (i.e., until the introduction of levodopa), trihexyphenidyl and its cousins were the chief anti-Parkinson drugs in common use. But, with the advent of levodopa, their use gradually declined. We rarely use these agents today in ordinary Parkinson's disease except when tremor is the predominant and functionally disabling symptom and is not responsive to other drugs. They are more useful in treating drug-induced parkinsonism. In contrast to levodopa, these drugs can reverse the parkinsonism induced by tranquilizer drugs.

Trihexyphenidyl is available in white 2- and 5-mg scored tablets and in a blue 5-mg slow-release capsule. We usually start at a low dose (one-half tablet once or twice a day) and increase it slowly. The 2-mg scored tablet may be broken in half, and 1 mg taken at each dose. If the 2-mg tablet is well tolerated, the dose may be increased to one 5-mg tablet three times daily. More than 15 mg daily is rarely helpful in Parkinson's disease. Indeed, most patients cannot tolerate larger doses.

Another synthetic anticholinergic agent widely used in treating parkinsonism is benztropine mesylate (Cogentin, Merck & Co., Inc.). The molecular structure of this drug is closely patterned after that of atropine, hence the *tropine* in its generic name. It is somewhat more potent than trihexyphenidyl and is, consequently, made in smaller dosage forms: 0.5-, 1-, and 2-mg tablets. It is also available, as is biperiden (Akineton), in a liquid form for injection with a hypodermic needle. It is used to treat parkinsonism and other, similar reactions to tranquilizer drugs. A single injection can terminate the tranquilizer reaction within minutes.

Many tricyclic antidepressants (TCA) such as amitriptyline (Elavil, Zeneca Pharmaceuticals) or imipramine (Tofranil, Novartis Pharmaceuticals Corporation) also have anticholinergic activity, but this is usually not strong enough to benefit tremor.

ANTIHISTAMINES

Atropine was once widely used in the treatment of asthma. The search for a drug that would have atropine's effect in asthma and other allergies but not its anticholinergic effects led to the development of the drug diphenhydramine (Benadryl, Warner–Lambert Consumer Healthcare, Morris Plains, NJ, U.S.A.). Introduced around 1946, this drug proved highly successful and was soon widely used in the treatment of hay fever, asthma, and many other allergies. Its success led to the introduction of many related drugs for the treatment of allergies. Their beneficial effect is thought to be due to their ability to block the action of the natural substance *histamine* formed in the body during allergic reactions; these drugs are thus classified as *antihistamines*. Some of these, notably diphenhydramine, were accidentally found to have some effect on the symptoms of Parkinson's disease. Although diphenhydramine itself has not been marketed and advertised to physicians as an anti-Parkinson drug, it has, nonetheless, been widely used in treating parkinsonism. The dosage required to affect parkinsonian symptoms is 50 mg two to four times daily.

Many other antihistamines not normally thought of as anti-Parkinson drugs, nevertheless, affect parkinsonian symptoms. The reason antihistamines may be helpful in parkinsonism has nothing to do with their properties as antihistamines; instead it is the fact that all have some anticholinergic properties. Trihexyphenidyl is approximately 25 times more potent an anticholinergic agent than is diphenhydramine, and so the latter is used in dosages 25 times as great. Thus 50 mg of diphenhydramine is as effective in relieving parkinsonian symptoms as 2 mg of trihexyphenidyl. Any drug having some anticholinergic effect also has some anti-Parkinson effect.

CHOLINERGIC DRUGS

There are drugs that enhance or imitate the action in the nervous system of the chemical messenger acetylcholine. Naturally, these are called *cholinergic drugs*. It is an interesting fact that cholinergic drugs exacerbate the symptoms of parkinsonism! For example, injection of a small dose of the drug physostigmine

(Antilirium, Forest Pharmaceuticals Inc., St. Louis, MO, U.S.A.), which enhances the action of acetylcholine in the brain, produces within minutes a marked increase in the tremor, rigidity, and other symptoms of parkinsonism. This effect subsides spontaneously within about 45 minutes.

It is clearly a good idea for Parkinson patients to avoid cholinergic drugs. In practice, however, very few cholinergic drugs are used, and the likelihood of a patient encountering one inadvertently (i.e., one that can get into the brain and exacerbate parkinsonian symptoms) is quite remote. Cholinergic drugs are being used more extensively in medical practice. Pilocarpine is used in the form of eye-drops to treat glaucoma; and bethanechol (Urecholine, Merck & Co. Inc.) is used to stimulate the bladder. These drugs do not affect parkinsonian symptoms. The manufacturer of bethanechol lists parkinsonism in the prescribing directions as a condition in which this drug should not be used. However, we have often used it to stimulate sluggish bladders of Parkinson patients and have rarely seen an adverse effect on the parkinsonian symptoms. It is highly unlikely that bethanechol in the doses ordinarily used will have an effect on the Parkinson state. Recently, several new cholinergic drugs [e.g., tacrine (Cognex, Parke–Davis, Morris Plains, NJ, U.S.A.), donepezil (Aricept, Eisai Inc., Teaneck, NJ, U.S.A.), and rivastigmine (Exelon, Novartis Pharmaceuticals Corporation)] have been introduced as treatment for Alzheimer's disease. They may partially correct the forgetfulness that is a common symptom of that condition. These drugs generally should not be given to Parkinson patients, since they have the potential to worsen the Parkinson symptoms. We have seen a few patients, however, who say that their memory improved on these drugs without worsening the Parkinson motor symptoms.

ANTICHOLINERGIC DRUG INTOXICATION

All the drugs discussed in this chapter depend on their anticholinergic properties for their usefulness in treating parkinsonism; that is, they block the action of the chemical messenger acetylcholine in the brain. By the same token, their side effects are due to the same mechanism. Blocking acetylcholine too severely produces undesirable effects, and the side effects are essentially the same with all the anticholinergic drugs. There is a common pattern that we term *anticholinergic intoxication*.

The most common side effects are dryness of the mouth, blurring of near vision, constipation, and weakening of the bladder. In addition, there is a whole range of mental side effects. Dryness of the mouth is due to a reduced flow of saliva. The saliva is also thicker and harder to swallow. The throat and nose may feel dry. The symptom is most marked when first starting treatment with anticholinergics. Partial tolerance develops within a few weeks, and most patients find it only a minor nuisance with continuing treatment. Some seek relief by sucking on bitter lemon candies or other hard sweets.

Blurring of near vision is due to the fact that anticholinergic drugs tend to diminish the action of the fine muscle in the eye that changes the shape of the lens to focus on near objects. Normally, the eye has universal focus for everything more than 18 inches away. To get a sharp view of objects at closer range, it is necessary to change the shape of the lens of the eye. This change is called "accommodation." Ophthalmologists regularly put drops of atropine or a synthetic anticholinergic in the eye for the purpose of "paralyzing accommodation," so that the optical properties of the eye can be tested precisely. Taking an anticholinergic drug by mouth produces the same effect, but to a lesser degree. For this reason, many patients notice difficulty in reading or doing close work when they first start on anticholinergic drugs. People normally have increasing difficulty with near vision after reaching middle age (called presbyopia). Age renders the individual more susceptible to this effect of anticholinergics. In addition, anticholinergics cause the pupil to open a bit more widely. This may also contribute to the blurring of near vision. Generally, the visual effect of the anticholinergics diminishes after a while. If it proves persistent, however, a new set of reading glasses can be obtained.

The tendency to widen or dilate the pupil may exacerbate glaucoma. Patients who have Parkinson's disease and glaucoma should be carefully checked by their eye doctor when treatment with anticholinergics is begun. If the glaucoma is under proper treatment or has been surgically corrected, there is usually no difficulty. The eye doctor can readily check the pressure of the eye to make sure that the treatment for the parkinsonism does not adversely affect the glaucoma.

Anticholinergic drugs typically slow the motor activity of the intestine. The waves of contraction, called peristalsis, are slowed. For this reason, many anticholinergic drugs are employed to treat disorders of the stomach and intestine; for example, the drug diphenoxylate–atropine sulfate (Lomotil, G. D. Searle & Co., Chicago, IL, U.S.A.) is commonly used to treat diarrhea. However, by the same token, the constipation of Parkinson's disease may be somewhat increased. This is rarely a serious problem, but if constipation is troublesome, it can be managed with stool softeners, dietary measures, bulking agents, mineral oil, or gentle laxatives.

A similar calming effect is exerted by anticholinergic drugs on the musculature of the urinary bladder. In a sense, these drugs sedate the bladder. This may be helpful to the patient troubled with urinary urgency who needs to get up several times during the night to void. An anticholinergic drug given at bedtime may help relieve this symptom. Indeed, the drug hyoscyamine [Cystospaz, PolyMedica Pharmaceuticals (U.S.A.), Inc., Woburn, MA, U.S.A.] one of the solanaceous alkaloids mentioned earlier, is commonly prescribed by urologists to control this symptom; others are oxybutynin chloride (Ditropan) and tolterodine (Detrol), which are synthetic anticholinergics. However, in the older male patient who has trouble due to an enlarged prostate gland obstructing the flow of urine, this calming effect can lead to urinary retention. Thus anticholinergic drugs are given with caution to patients who have symptoms of prostatic obstruction. The need to pass a catheter can usually be averted by using very small doses of the drug. It may, of course, be necessary to operate on the prostate. A specialist in urology should be consulted before symptoms of urinary obstruction reach a severe stage.

The mental effects of anticholinergic drugs are important and, in many ways, very interesting. The fact that ingestion of the leaves of jimsonweed, henbane, or deadly nightshade can cause mental disturbances has been known since ancient times. Abuse of these botanicals for psychedelic effects has been described repeatedly. Nearly every year one sees news reports of children becoming delirious after eating jimsonweed leaves. The symptoms include confusion, agitation, hallucinations, stupor, and in severe intoxication, coma. The symptoms subside within a day or two except for amnesia for the episode.

The first and most common mental side effect noticeable in patients being treated with any anticholinergic drug is forgetfulness, mainly for recent events. Patients may forget where they left their glasses a minute ago or what they went to buy at the corner store. Occasionally, mild confusion then appears. Visual illusions are especially frequent. Familiar objects may be mistaken for something else. The patient may mention seeing worms on the floor, misinterpreting a pattern design in the flooring because it seems to move. Spectral illusions, generally of a benign if not pleasing character, are experienced. There may be hallucinations of people or animals roaming about the house. Most commonly, there seem to be complex scenes, such as a group of people wandering about, having a party. They may be smaller than normal and seem to go about their business without disturbing the patient. Patients may experience these visions for long periods of time but are afraid to mention them to anyone for fear of being thought "crazy." Finally, however, in a moment of confusion, the patient reacts to these illusions. Some patients angrily order the strangers out of the house, accuse them of stealing, or call the police to chase them away. At this point, the patient's family, not having previously noticed anything out of the ordinary, become alarmed. These disturbances usually disappear if the dosage of the anticholinergic drug is reduced. The physician should check to see if these disturbances followed a change in medication or the addition of a new drug. A patient who has been doing well on a standard dose of, say, trihexyphenidyl may suddenly develop such mental disturbances when another drug is added. For example, the patient may have taken an antihistamine because of hay fever symptoms. The anticholinergic properties of the antihistamine added to the anticholinergic properties of trihexyphenidyl then carried the patient over the threshold into a mild state of anticholinergic intoxication. Usually, the disturbance subsides within a day or so after the new drug is discontinued. If there has been no change of medication, the patient's drug regimen may be revised downward. Usually, it is not a good idea to give a tranquilizer unless there is severe agitation. Many of the commonly used major tranquilizers also have some anticholinergic properties, and so the confusion and hallucinations may be increased even if the agitation is controlled for a few hours.

Some patients are very sensitive to the toxic mental effects of the anticholinergic drugs and cannot tolerate any of them, not even very mild ones such as the antihistamines. A few patients develop these mental reactions even after the mildest sleep medications. Rarely, a patient experiences these disturbances spontaneously, on no treatment at all. There is probably something inherent to Parkinson's disease that makes one susceptible to these mental disturbances (see the section on diffuse Lewy body disease in Chapter 1).

Another effect of the anticholinergic drugs that may be good or bad, depending on the circumstances, is the tendency to reduce sweating. Excessive sweating, sometimes occurring irregularly in bursts, is an occasional symptom of Parkinson's disease. Anticholinergic drugs can diminish this excessive perspiration, sometimes not as much as desired and sometimes too much. We depend on sweating to cool our bodies in warm weather. The brain controls the amount of sweat we produce, thereby regulating body temperature. Anticholinergic drugs may impair this regulation, and in warm weather fever and even coma may result. This is a rare occurrence today but was a familiar problem years ago when large doses of atropine were commonly used in treating parkinsonism.

ADVERSE REACTIONS

Adverse reactions have been very rare with the anticholinergic drugs. We have never seen one, but there are reports in medical journals of isolated instances of allergic skin rashes, inflammation of the liver, and a rare toxic effect on the bone marrow resulting in a lack of white blood corpuscles.

AMANTADINE

A Parkinson's disease patient of the late Dr. Robert Schwab reported that while taking the drug amantadine (Symmetrel, Endo Laboratories, Chadds Ford, PA, U.S.A.) as protection against catching the flu she felt better. This drug had been developed as an antiviral agent and is protective against the flu virus. Dr. Schwab confirmed this observation and then treated other Parkinson patients with amantadine, finding that many of these patients looked and felt better while taking the drug. Other doctors also tried amantadine in their Parkinson patients and corroborated Dr. Schwab's report.

Amantadine does indeed possess some property that partially alleviates the symptoms of Parkinson's disease. Its side effect—blurred vision, constipation, mental confusion, dryness of the mouth—suggest that it acts as an anticholinergic drug. However, laboratory studies failed to show a direct acetylcholine blocking effect. It had been reported that amantadine enhances the function of dopamine nerve cells, and it was thought that it mimicked the effects of L-dopa, the precursor of dopamine. However, this effect has only been shown in test tube experiments, with amounts of the drug far greater than the dosages that can be used in humans. Thus although it is still often referred to as a "dopaminergic" drug, we do not agree that amantadine can be so classified. Scientists have found that it indirectly blocks the action of acetylcholine. Thus we consider one of the actions of amantadine to be that of an anticholinergic agent.

Recently, Dr. Thomas Chase and his colleagues at the National Institutes of Health have noted that amantadine in high doses reduces levodopa-induced involuntary movements. This effect is thought to be mediated by blocking receptors in the brain for *N*-methyl-D-aspartate (NMDA). Regulation of NMDA or similar substances may play a role in future treatments of Parkinson's disease.

Amantadine is available in a 100-mg capsule. The normal dose is one capsule two or three times daily, although some patients may take as many as four, particularly if it is being used to decrease involuntary movements. It is also available in a liquid solution. Since it may augment the side effects of anticholinergic drugs such as trihexyphenidyl and cause confusion or hallucinations, care is usually taken to change doses slowly when the two drugs are used simultaneously. We rarely use both drugs together.

A unique and unusual side effect of amantadine is the appearance of a curious faint purplish mottling of the skin of the legs and sometimes the arms due to blood pooling in small veins in the skin. It usually appears only after several months and may take 1 to 2 months to subside after the drug is stopped. This unusual side effect is apparently harmless. It is called *livido reticularis* (Fig. 8). Sometimes the purplish mottling is accompanied by swelling of the feet and ankles due to the accumulation of water in the soft tissues. The medical term for this accumulation of water is *edema*. Although it may be ungainly and worrisome, this too appears to be harmless and disappears when amantadine is discontinued.

Another curious property of amantadine is that it may lose its effectiveness after several months. However, if the patient stops taking the drug for a while and

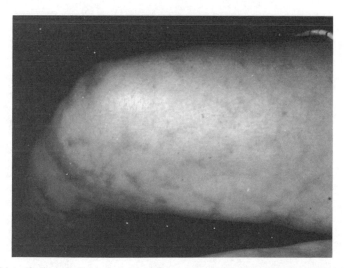

FIG. 8. Livido reticularis is the purplish mottling of the skin on the leg of a patient treated with amantadine.

then uses it again, it usually regains its effectiveness. Although this phenomenon occurs in only some patients, it is worthwhile to determine whether amantadine is still effective when a patient has been taking it for some time. We often advise our patients in such circumstances to discontinue the drug for a week or so. If there is no change and the patient does not feel worse, there seems no point in taking it again. It may then be discontinued completely and tried again after a month or two. On the other hand, if the patient is definitely worse after stopping the amantadine, drug treatment should be promptly resumed because it is clear that the drug is worth taking.

7

From L-Dopa to Dopamine

What drug can make a withered palsy cease to shake?

"The Two Voices," Alfred Tennyson

L-Dopa is the most effective substance currently available for the treatment of Parkinson's disease. Its full chemical name is l-3,4-dihydroxyphenylalanine. Chemists have for many years abbreviated this cumbersome name to the simpler *dopa"* or L-*dopa*. Persons not versed in the language of chemistry sometimes fear that the name *dopa* has a more sinister meaning. Patients often ask if the drug L-dopa contains "dope." Many wonder if it is a Spanish drug, for they understand L-dopa to be El Dopa. Others inquire about the ingredients of L-dopa.

L-Dopa is, in fact, merely a simple chemical substance occurring in nature in both animals and plants. It is not a mixture of ingredients but a single, rather simple molecule belonging to a class of substances known to chemists as amino acids and composed of atoms of carbon, hydrogen, oxygen, and nitrogen. The arrangement of these atoms in the dopa molecule is shown in Fig. 9. Its shape in three-dimensional space is such that the dopa molecule can exist in two forms, each the mirror image of the other, just as the right hand is the mirror image of the left. The bones and ligaments of both hands are connected in exactly the same way, yet the two hands are not exactly the same in three-dimensional space; they cannot fit in the same glove. The two forms of the dopa molecule are designated the levo form (from the Latin *laevo*, meaning "left") and the dextro form (from the Latin prefix *dexter*, meaning "right")—or more simply, the L- and D-forms.

Many molecules exist in duplicate mirror forms, such as L-glucose and D-glucose, L-amphetamine and D-amphetamine, L-ryptophan and D-tryptophan, and so on. Just as your right hand cannot fit in a left-hand glove, so the L-forms of these molecules cannot fit in the same spaces as the D-forms. Consequently, the two forms of these molecules often have different physical properties, form crystals of different shapes, and behave differently in the biological world. It is a remarkable fact that plants and animals make and use only the L-forms! Only the L-form

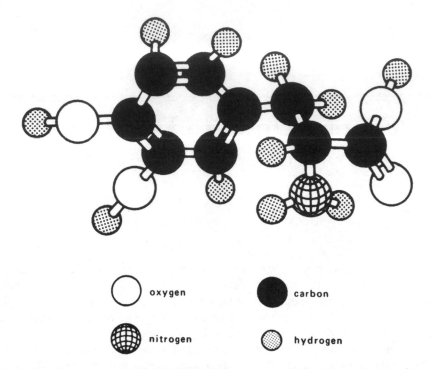

FIG. 9. Model of the dopa molecule. The nitrogen and its attached hydrogen atom form an amine group, which confers the chemical properties of an alkali on the molecule. The group at the far right end of the molecule—consisting of a carbon atom holding an oxygen atom with two arms (or bonds) and an oxygen–hydrogen combination with one bond—is called a *carboxyl group*. This confers the properties of an acid on the molecule. Dopa is thus an amino acid. Removal of the carboxyl group—a step called decarboxylation and controlled by an enzyme aptly enough called a *decarboxylase*—converts the dopa molecule to a dopamine molecule.

of dopa is found in nature, and only the L-form is effective in treating Parkinson's disease. The D-form is inert!

L-Dopa was first discovered in 1908 in the broad bean or fava bean (*Vicia faba*) used in Mediterranean cooking. It is also present in the velvet bean (*Mucuna pruriens*), the locoweed, and certain other related legumes. Botanists have suggested that L-dopa serves to protect the plants from insects.

L-Dopa also occurs in the animal kingdom, where it plays an important role as an intermediate substance in the metabolism of adrenaline, the hormone secreted into the circulation by the adrenal gland to prepare the body for "fight or flight" in an emergency. The adrenal gland makes adrenaline in a series of chemical reactions that begin with the amino acid tyrosine, an ingredient of our diet. Tyrosine is found mainly in the proteins we eat every day. An ordinary American hamburger, for example, contains 1 to 2 g of tyrosine. When we eat a hamburger or other meat, the protein molecules in it are broken down during digestion to simpler molecules called peptides. These, in turn, are further broken down into their component amino acids. After being absorbed by the intestines, the amino acids are transported in the blood first to the liver and then to other organs throughout the body. Most of the tyrosine we absorb from our daily diet is used to build new protein. A very small proportion is taken up from the circulation by the cells of the adrenal gland. There it is immediately converted by a single molecular rearrangement to L-dopa. L-Dopa, in turn, is promptly changed into dopamine via another chemical reaction. In turn, dopamine is changed into norepinephrine, and in the final step in this metabolic pathway noradrenaline is converted into adrenaline. The adrenaline is then stored by the cells of the adrenal gland in little packets, which can be seen under the electron microscope, until such time as the gland receives a signal from the nervous system to release it into the bloodstream.

This pathway of sequential chemical reactions occurs in exactly the same way in the substantia nigra of the brain. Here, however, the process ends with the formation of dopamine. The dopamine is then stored in the ends of the fibers of substantia nigra cells. These fibers spread throughout the corpus striatum, and the dopamine stored there is released to function as a chemical messenger at the dopamine receptors located on the nerve cells in the striatum. In other areas of the nervous system (e.g., in the sympathetic nerves), the process ends with the formation of noradrenaline.

The step from tyrosine to dopa in the adrenal gland and the brain is strictly controlled and is called a "rate-limiting" step. Feeding large amounts of tyrosine does not result in the formation of larger amounts of dopamine or of noradrenaline or adrenaline. This is not surprising. If it were not so, every time we ate a lot of protein we would have too much adrenaline in our systems. However, the step from L-dopa to dopamine is not subject to such control, and so it is possible to increase the amount of dopamine formed in the brain by feeding large amounts of L-dopa. Thus tyrosine has little effect in treating parkinsonism, whereas L-dopa is very effective. Essentially, L-dopa relieves the symptoms of parkinsonism by restoring brain dopamine at least partially to normal levels. L-dopa itself is inert. All its actions are due to the dopamine derived from it in the various organs of the body.

LEVODOPA TREATMENT

L-Dopa is the name employed by chemists to describe this interesting substance. However, L-dopa prepared for use as a drug is officially termed *levodopa*. This is the international generic name of the medicinal form of L-dopa. It is marketed, of course, under various trade names by different pharmaceutical firms.

Levodopa taken by mouth passes through the stomach into the duodenum and then to the upper and small intestine, where it is absorbed. The process of absorption takes place over a period of several hours. We can study this process by measuring (via chemical means) the amount of levodopa in the blood at various intervals after a dose is ingested. Measurements done on different patients or on the same patient on different days vary somewhat, but in general the level of levodopa in the blood (normally zero) gradually rises to a peak value approximately 30 minutes to 2 hours after a dose is taken by mouth, then gradually falls back to zero again within 4 to 6 hours. The results of such a study, plotted as a graph, are seen in Fig. 10.

From such studies a number of things have been found to influence the absorption of levodopa. One of the most important is the amount and type of food in the stomach. Solid food, especially food containing protein, delays the absorption of levodopa and may reduce the amount taken up in the circulation. Many patients are aware of this effect of food. They have observed that the relief of their symptoms is greater and comes on more rapidly when they take a dose of levodopa on an empty stomach than when they take it after a meal. Many have also noted that their usual dose may have little or no effect if taken after a hearty steak dinner. Patients on a low-protein diet need less levodopa to obtain the same result they experience with higher doses on a regular diet.

If the stomach is excessively acid, it empties into the duodenum more slowly, and consequently the absorption of levodopa is delayed. In such circumstances,

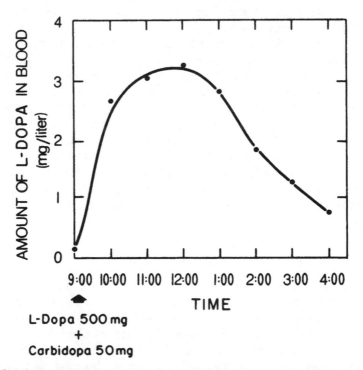

FIG. 10. Graph shows the amount of levodopa at various times in the blood of a patient after a single dose was administered at 9:00 a.m. Blood was then drawn from a vein each hour until 4:00 p.m. The highest blood level of levodopa was measured in the sample taken at 12:00 noon.

taking some milk or an antacid tablet with the levodopa improves the absorption of levodopa. Some patients report that chewing the levodopa tablet rather than swallowing it provides faster relief of their symptoms. They use this trick for a "booster" effect, usually with supplementary midafternoon doses. Levodopa, however, is not absorbed from the mouth.

Once absorbed into the circulation, levodopa travels throughout the entire body. A large proportion of the dose taken by mouth ends up in muscles, fat stores, the liver, skin, kidney, and other organs. Most of it is rapidly converted to dopamine in the blood vessels in the various organs, especially the kidney, and is excreted in the urine in the form of various inactive substances.

Only a very small proportion of the oral dose of levodopa, probably less than 1%, ultimately penetrates the brain. There it is selectively taken up by the dopamine nerve cells of the substantia nigra and possibly by other cells and then converted to dopamine. In this manner the brain stores of dopamine may be at least partially replenished.

Of course, some time is required for the levodopa to leave the bloodstream, cross the walls of the blood vessels, enter the brain, and reach the dopamine cells, where it may then be converted to dopamine. Animal studies indicate that this delay is usually 15 to 30 minutes. Thus, if the peak blood level of levodopa is reached 1 hour after ingestion, the peak brain level of dopamine must be reached approximately 1 hour and 15 minutes to 1 hour and 30 minutes after ingestion. Of course, some effects may begin to be felt 20 to 30 minutes after taking a dose of levodopa by mouth, but the full effect does not occur until at least an hour and a half later. The newly formed dopamine in the brain joins the dopamine formed in the normal manner from tyrosine as just described. In this way, brain dopamine stores are replenished, and the symptoms of parkinsonism are correspondingly diminished. In the earlier stages of Parkinson's disease, dopamine storage is adequate and patients get a smooth response by taking two or three levodopa tablets per day. As storage capacity decreases, motor fluctuations begin to occur (see Motor Fluctuations, below).

Levodopa treatment, however, is not a cure. As far as we know, it does not affect the basic disease process—whatever it may be—responsible for the dysfunction of the brain's dopamine cells or bring back those that may have deteriorated. It merely helps the dopamine nerve cells make dopamine more readily. Apparently, it helps the cells function better despite their illness. Levodopa treatment is thus a symptomatic treatment. That is, it is a treatment that can relieve symptoms without correcting the underlying or primary cause. It may also be considered a replacement therapy (i.e., a treatment based on replacing a substance essential to the body's economy that is deficient). The same may be said of other forms of treatment in modern medicine: thyroid hormone treatment for hypothyroidism, for example, or insulin treatment for diabetes. In diabetes mellitus, there is a deficiency of insulin, the hormone that regulates sugar metabolism throughout the body. The diabetic patient may be given insulin by injection to provide the body with the insulin it needs but cannot make itself in sufficient amounts. In this way, the disturbance in sugar metabolism that causes so much of the trouble in diabetes can be corrected. However, insulin does not cure diabetes. It does not correct the basic disease—whatever it is—and restore the body's ability to make proper amounts of insulin.

When levodopa treatment is first begun, the patient feels a gradual improvement over a period of several days. An appreciable response is usually achieved within 3 to 5 days, but further improvement builds up more slowly over the subsequent weeks. The full effect of treatment may not be apparent for 2 to 3 months of continuing treatment. Most patients are not aware of the effect of each individual dose. Nor are they aware of any definite change if they miss a given dose. If a dose is missed inadvertently, there is little point in trying to make up the lost dose by taking more pills the next time the medicine is due. When treatment is stopped for any reason, the parkinsonian symptoms return gradually over a period of several days. Little change may be noted the first day. Definite change is experienced the second day after stopping treatment and still more the third and fourth days. Most of the benefit of levodopa treatment is lost by the fourth or fifth days, but it may take 1 to 2 weeks before the effect of levodopa is completely gone. The slowness of the response to treatment and the long duration of the response when treatment is stopped indicate that in most patients the brain is able to store dopamine for some period of time, and that to fill up the dopamine stores may require several months of continuing treatment. It is as if a large reservoir is being filled through a small opening with a small bucket. Many buckets and some time are required to fill the reservoir to its full capacity.

MOTOR FLUCTUATIONS

Some patients after a period of years of treatment feel the effect of each dose of levodopa. They can tell when a given dose begins to work, to diminish their symptoms. They can also tell when the effect of a given dose wears off. Such patients may also experience some return of their parkinsonian symptoms in the morning, before the first dose of the day. They seem to have lost the "sleep benefit" that most patients receive. Apparently, the levodopa effect wears off overnight, presumably because the dopamine reserves diminished during the long interval between the last dose at night and the first dose the following morning. In other words, these patients do not have a long enough response to levodopa to maintain full control of their symptoms for a long time. They are said to have primarily a short-duration response, which may reflect a decreased capacity to store dopamine. The reservoir is leaky, or it has become smaller.

Patients who note that the effectiveness of each dose begins to wear off after 3 to 4 hours or more may benefit from newer controlled-release preparations of levodopa (Sinemet CR or Madopar HBS). These formulations contain the same ingredients as standard tablets but are designed to release levodopa more slowly. They therefore provide steadier concentrations of dopamine to the basal ganglia over a longer time period, and their effectiveness does not depend on the ability of the brain to store dopamine. Patients with mild or moderate fluctuations taking controlled-release levodopa usually experience fewer wearing-off symptoms and can often take fewer doses each day.

In a small percentage of patients, the response to levodopa appears to be chiefly of the short-duration variety. These patients fluctuate markedly from a state of parkinsonism to a state of normal movement and back again several times a day. The change from one state to the other may take place quite rapidly. Some patients have said that it felt as if an electric switch had been turned on or off. For this reason this phenomenon has been termed the *on–off* effect. The fluctuations can be smoothed out to some extent by adjusting the dosage schedule to the duration of the individual patient's response. Thus, instead of taking levodopa only three or four times daily as is usual, such a patient might take it every 3 hours—or even every 2 hours—throughout the day. It is rarely worthwhile to take levodopa more frequently than every 2 hours. The precise timing can be very important and must be carefully worked out, by trial and error, in each patient. Generally, results are best if the patient follows a definite schedule strictly "by the clock" and works closely with the doctor to develop the most appropriate schedule. Some patients with this on–off problem are able to judge sufficiently in advance when an "off" phase is coming and so take their levodopa dose when they feel the need. However, in our experience, most patients who self-regulate their dosage schedules according to their own subjective feeling do poorly. They tend to overdose themselves and become confused about how much to take and when to take it. Often they cannot tell whether their symptoms at any one time are due to overdosage or underdosage and fail to distinguish the symptoms of parkinsonism from the side effects of levodopa.

NAUSEA AND VOMITING

Dopamine formed from taking the medication levodopa accumulates not only in the corpus striatum but in other brain areas as well. This may be all to the good, but it may also give rise to undesired side effects. A major side effect when levodopa therapy was first being developed was nausea and vomiting. We have since learned to lessen this side effect, and it is no longer the problem it was. Moreover, levodopa is now usually given in combination with an enzyme-inhibitor drug, either carbidopa or benserazide, that prevents the conversion of levodopa to dopamine throughout the body *except* in the brain. A major benefit of this combination treatment is a marked decrease in the frequency and severity of nausea and vomiting. Nevertheless, since nausea and vomiting still occasionally occur even with the combination treatment, we should consider in some detail the mechanism of this unpleasant side effect and the methods of dealing with it that proved useful when only levodopa was available. We will discuss this again in the section on enzyme-inhibitor drugs.

There is a specialized area known as the area postrema, located in the brainstem near the junction of the brain and the spinal cord. (See Fig. 2 in Chapter 1.) This is the vomiting center. It contains nerve cells whose task is to detect toxins or poisons in the circulation and to prevent further absorption of such substances by provoking the stomach to empty its contents to throw out the offending material.

The vomiting center is sensitive to levodopa, adrenaline, and many other substances. Apparently, it regards levodopa, an unusual substance to find in the circulation, as an offensive material to be thrown out. As the blood level of levodopa rises approximately 30 minutes after a dose, the vomiting center may be activated. It can also be activated when levodopa is given by direct injection into the bloodstream through a vein. The vomiting induced by levodopa is not due to irritation of the stomach itself, but this makes little difference to the patient who experiences it. First, there is a general discomfort, a sense of weakness, and a disinterest in eating. If activation of the center is more marked, there is a metallic taste in the mouth, nausea, and dizziness. These symptoms may subside after a half hour or so, especially if the patient lies down. If the activation is sufficient, vomiting occurs even if there is nothing in the stomach. The vomiting usually comes very suddenly and is over very quickly, and the patient usually feels better soon afterward.

Unfortunately, the dose of levodopa required to relieve the symptoms of parkinsonism is more than enough to activate the vomiting center in most persons. There are exceptions, of course. We have seen patients who took full doses of levodopa alone from the first day of treatment and never felt any nausea. At the other extreme there are patients who never tolerate full doses of levodopa and fail to develop tolerance even after many months. In the early experiments with levodopa, this state of affairs was a major obstacle to the development of an effective means of using levodopa to treat parkinsonism. However, two facts about the vomiting center make it possible to overcome this problem in most patients.

The first of these is that repeated exposure to levodopa causes the vomiting center to gradually become accustomed to its presence so that the center no longer responds to it. The second is that the vomiting center is most likely to react when the blood level of dopa is rising rapidly; that is, when the levodopa taken by mouth is absorbed especially well. Thus it is possible to "tame" the vomiting center by starting treatment with small doses of levodopa and by taking levodopa only after meals to slow its absorption. In practice, the major problem has been with breakfast. Many people do not eat much for breakfast—a glass of orange juice, a cup of coffee, and toast. That is not enough to slow the absorption of levodopa. In fact, the caffeine in coffee may help levodopa activate the vomiting center.

Patients taking their first doses of levodopa after such a small breakfast (or nonbreakfast) are especially apt to feel at least some nausea or loss of interest in food. As lunchtime rolls around a few hours later, they may still be disinclined to eat and thus content themselves with a cup of coffee for lunch. This time, the vomiting center, still disturbed by the morning dose of levodopa, may react more violently and vomiting results. In the days before the current formulations of levodopa were available, the answers to this problem were threefold: (a) make sure that breakfast includes some solid food, preferably food containing protein; (b) change to decaffeinated coffee or tea; and (c) if necessary, reduce the morning dose of levodopa. If the patient still reacted with nausea and vomiting after trying these measures, some antivomiting drug was tried. Unfortunately, the most effective antivomiting drugs antagonize levodopa. They not only block the activation of the vomiting center by levodopa but also prevent the relief of parkinsonism. So treatment had to rely on milder antivomiting drugs, and these often did the trick. They included diphenidol (Vontrol, SmithKline Beecham) and trimethobenzamide (Tigan, Roberts Pharmaceutical Corporation, Eatontown, NJ, U.S.A.). The old anti-Parkinson drugs such as trihexyphenidyl (Artane) and even the common antihistamine diphenhydramine hydrochloride (Benadryl) also give some protection against the activation of the vomiting center. Thus, when beginning levodopa treatment, a patient already taking trihexyphenidyl or a drug of that class was continued on it during the initial period of levodopa treatment.

The more slowly the dose of levodopa is raised, the less likely it is that nausea and vomiting will occur. Normally, it seems to take 3 to 6 months to develop full tolerance to the action of levodopa on the vomiting center. Thus, the patient should not be in too great a hurry to enjoy the good effects of levodopa in full measure. Both patient and physician should be willing to wait a few months before reaching the ultimate dosage schedule. Of course, personal tolerance levels vary considerably. Some patients never experience even the slightest nausea, whereas others are unable to develop a sufficient tolerance to reach effective doses of levodopa even after several years.

INVOLUNTARY MOVEMENTS (DYSKINESIAS)

The most common side effect of levodopa treatment is the production of various involuntary movements. These include twitches, jerks, nods, gestures, twisting or writhing movements, or simple restlessness. The neurologic term for these movements is *dyskinesia*. These movements can be so minimal as to be barely perceptible. When they are somewhat more obvious but still very mild, they seem to be no more than restlessness or fidgetiness. Usually, patients are not aware of them until they become at least mild in magnitude. Patients usually do not mind the movements even when they are quite obvious. When severe, they become tiring and cause clumsiness and awkwardness. The rapid, dancelike movements are called *chorea*. Slow, twisting movements, sustained postures, and muscle cramps are called *dystonia*. The most common movements appear at higher doses of levodopa and usually occur only for a brief period, 1 to 2 hours after a dose, a time when the brain levels of dopamine are highest. This is called *peak-dose dyskinesia*.

The movements can be abolished by drugs that block the action of dopamine (e.g., the major tranquilizers). However, these drugs also block the desired effects of levodopa and thus are helpful only in rare emergency situations to treat overdosage with levodopa. Many treatments have been tried in the hope of finding a way of preventing the movements without also preventing the relief of parkinsonian symptoms. Thus far no entirely effective means of doing this has been found. Switching from standard levodopa to a controlled-release preparation may help to some extent because the longer-acting formulations are also designed to produce lower peak concentrations of brain dopamine As already mentioned, high doses of amantadine may reduce dyskinesias. In many patients, however, the only way of handling the problem is to lower the dosage of levodopa. Unfortunately, many patients then have some recurrence of their parkinsonism. Most patients prefer a compromise in which some movements are present and better relief of the parkinsonism is obtained. This dilemma is the major shortcoming of levodopa therapy.

In many ways chorea and parkinsonism are opposites. In chorea there is excessive bodily movement, whereas in parkinsonism there is too little bodily movement. In chorea the muscles are loose and floppy; in parkinsonism they are stiff and rigid. Drugs that cause parkinsonism are useful in treating chorea. The converse, it seems, is also true: Levodopa, a drug that can cause chorea, is useful in treating parkinsonism. Thus the production of chorealike movements in a Parkinson patient reflects an overcorrection of the parkinsonism and an excessive amount of dopamine in the brain at the precise moment the movements are present. A half hour later, when the movements cease, the brain dopamine level can be presumed to have decreased to a more desirable range.

Frankly, the involuntary movements are a normal, though undesirable, effect of levodopa in Parkinson patients that merely reflects the dosage. Curiously, levodopa does not induce these involuntary movements so readily in patients with other disorders or in normal volunteers. Parkinsonian patients are more susceptible than other people to the chorea-inducing effect of levodopa. Other drugs that alleviate parkinsonism can also induce involuntary movements, although to a lesser extent. Of course, these other drugs are also less effective in relieving the symptoms of parkinsonism. It seems then that the involuntary movements are due not only to the drug but also to something at work in the brain of Parkinson's disease patients. Just what that something may be is unknown. It seems reasonable to suspect that certain changes in the brain dopamine receptors that occur to compensate for the long-standing depletion of dopamine may be responsible.

The brain is somehow able to compensate for a great loss of dopamine for a very long time. How does it do this? One way seems to be to increase the rate at which dopamine is formed, perhaps to correct for the decreased capacity to store it. Another way the brain may compensate seems to be to increase its sensitivity to the actions of dopamine so that a smaller amount may provoke the same response. The brain cells that normally receive and respond to dopamine may thus become supersensitive to it and adapt to the diminished amount of their chemical messenger. Then, when dopamine becomes available again in normal amounts (when the patient starts taking levodopa), these cells respond in an exaggerated manner and the patient experiences dyskinesias (an increase in movement). It also seems probable that other nerve cells that do not normally process levodopa can convert it to dopamine, but they may release it inappropriately at the wrong times in response to the wrong signals and deliver it to unusual places. These adaptations do not seem to be reversed when levodopa therapy is begun. The involuntary movements do not diminish over time with continued treatment. No tolerance to this side effect appears to develop.

MENTAL EFFECTS OF LEVODOPA

Many patients describe a feeling of being more alert after first starting levodopa treatment. They appear more attentive and more spontaneous in their activity. They become more talkative, and they seem to have more initiative and to take more interest in the world around them. Some also complain of a feeling of nervousness, of an inner restlessness, or even "jitteriness." They may also have trouble sleeping at night. These effects are somewhat reminiscent of the effects of amphetamine and related drugs often given to combat drowsiness. This is not surprising because amphetamine works in the brain by activating the normal dopamine cells. Essentially, amphetamine causes these cells to release more dopamine than they normally would in the course of their usual traffic with other nerve cells. The actions of amphetamine can be blocked by drugs that block the action of dopamine. Usually, the nervousness, restlessness, and insomnia subside after a few weeks of continuing treatment.

Another, similar activating effect occasionally experienced by patients is vivid dreaming. They may not have dreamed in years, but after starting levodopa treatment they again enjoy dreaming. Usually, this is pleasant, but excessively vivid dreams may be distressing; rarely, they are nightmares. The simplest way of dealing with this problem is to avoid taking a bedtime dose of levodopa or to make the bedtime dose somewhat smaller. This effect also tends to diminish in time with continued treatment.

It is often difficult to tell whether a change in behavior after starting levodopa treatment is an improvement or a side effect. The patient who finds he or she has more energy and can resume doing many things around the house that had been turned over to others is improved. However, the spouse and family may complain that the patient is too "bossy," "stubborn," or "demanding." In some cases, it seems that the family resents the patient reasserting a former dominance, whereas at other times it is clear that a personality change has indeed occurred.

Increased sexual interest and activity have been described as a side effect. The increased interest is evident in a number of patients. In most, it has been a partial recovery toward normal, although in some the increased sexual activity seemed excessive and inappropriate. Most patients, however, experience no change in libido. Some years ago, the alleged effect of levodopa on sexual life attracted the interest of the press. Many of our patients who read the newspaper reports humorously asked what had been left out of their pills!

Rarely, levodopa seems to induce a hyperactive behavior in which the patient becomes agitated or "nervous," attempts too many projects, writes numerous letters, calls everyone he knows on the telephone, and plans ambitious undertakings. This manic or hypomanic behavior may occur episodically.

It is also rare for levodopa to provoke episodes of confused, irrational behavior. These may include visual hallucinations similar to those produced by the anticholinergic drugs. However, levodopa is much less prone to produce such effects than any of the other anti-Parkinson drugs. Patients who are especially sensitive to the hallucinogenic effect of these drugs should avoid all drugs, including sleep medications, antihistamines, cough suppressants, and so on, except levodopa. Even then the levodopa dosage should be adjusted very cautiously.

An increase in the dosage in an attempt to gain better control of the symptoms may initiate a train of mental symptoms in patients who have been on long-term treatment. Vivid dreams and nightmares lead to insomnia. Sleep medications prove to be of little help and insomnia persists. Agitation and confusion occur during the day, followed by visual hallucinations, which are often dreamlike in quality. This situation has been aptly termed the *dopa madness*. Reversing it requires reducing the dosage of levodopa or adding medications that block hallucinations (see Chapter 10). In severe cases, hospitalization may be needed.

Depression or melancholia is not uncommon among parkinsonian patients. Some physicians have reported that levodopa may exacerbate or provoke depression. Others have thought it might help alleviate depression; most feel it has no effect. In our experience, either effect may occur. Depression may be masked by the symptoms of parkinsonism, so that when the latter are relieved by levodopa treatment, the depression becomes apparent. Therefore, one should be alert to the possibility of depression. Effective treatment for depression is available and may be used in combination with levodopa therapy. Levodopa need not normally be discontinued. Usually, both conditions can be treated simultaneously. Drugs commonly used to treat depression such as imipramine (Tofranil) and amitriptyline (Elavil) may readily be used at the same time as levodopa and may even work better with levodopa than if used alone. Some of the newer antidepressants work by inhibiting uptake of the neurotransmitter serotonin, thereby making it more available for use by brain cells. Common drugs in this group that can be used effectively by patients with Parkinson's disease are fluoxetine (Prozac, Dista Products Co., Indianapolis, IN, U.S.A.), paroxetine (Paxil, SmithKline Beecham), and sertraline (Zoloft, Pfizer Inc.).

However, one group of drugs sometimes used to treat depression should never, under any circumstances, be given to a patient taking levodopa. This is the group of *monoamine oxidase (MAO) inhibitor* drugs. By blocking the action of the enzyme monoamine oxidase, these drugs turn off the body's normal mechanism for preventing excessive accumulation of dopamine, adrenaline, and noradrenaline. Levodopa can be metabolized to all three of these substances, and so they accumulate very rapidly in abnormal amounts in the body if levodopa and a

MAO inhibitor drug are taken together. The results are similar to the effects of an overdose of adrenaline. The heart pounds rapidly, the blood pressure shoots up very high, and palpitations, shortness of breath, nausea, vomiting, severe headaches, agitation, convulsions, and coma may result. There is a serious possibility of provoking a heart attack or a cerebral hemorrhage. Similar reactions can occur when a MAO inhibitor is combined with a variety of other drugs, such as amphetamine, and even with certain foods, especially cheddar cheese and certain wines. In fact, since this reaction was first noted in patients who ate cheese while being treated with a MAO inhibitor, it has been called the *cheese reaction.* The MAO inhibitor drugs in current use include pargyline (Eutonyl, Abbott Laboratories, North Chicago, IL, U.S.A.), phenelzine (Nardil, Parke–Davis), and tranylcypromine (Parnate, SmithKline Beecham).

LOW BLOOD PRESSURE

Levodopa also accumulates in other parts of the nervous system. It is believed to enter sympathetic nerves, which control the heart and blood vessels throughout the body. In these nerves, levodopa simply enters the normal metabolic pathway for the formation of adrenaline and noradrenaline. However, because it is present in unnatural amounts, it may interfere with the normal function of the sympathetic nervous system. The result may be episodes of rapid heartbeat (rapid pulse), which may be felt as palpitations. Elevation or depression of blood pressure may also occur. Indeed, dopamine is now employed as a drug in its own right to treat low blood pressure; it is injected by vein to raise blood pressure as an emergency measure in patients with very low blood pressure following serious injuries or major surgery, a condition known as *shock.* However, in patients taking levodopa, the blood pressure usually tends to decrease. In fact, in some patients it may fall to such low levels that such symptoms as faintness, dizziness, and lightheadedness result. Levodopa by mouth very rarely causes brief periods of high blood pressure. Low blood pressure is by far the most common side effect involving the circulatory system. A striking feature is that the blood pressure may be normal if measured in the lying or sitting position, only to fall when the patient stands up. This occurs because the blood pools in the legs. Normally, the sympathetic nervous system acts on the blood vessels to counter the effects of gravity and maintain a uniform flow of blood to the head. This is accomplished by constriction of blood vessels in the legs, which prevents accumulation of blood in the leg muscles. The sympathetic nervous system is somewhat impaired in some patients with Parkinson's disease. The effect of levodopa on these nerves may further impair their function, so that they may not be able to prevent the pooling of blood in the legs when the patient stands up.

This side effect of levodopa may be countered by several measures. A simple, frequently effective one is to administer salt tablets. Several tablets a day (containing 0.25 to 0.5 g of sodium chloride) suffice for most patients having this side effect. Another measure is to wear elastic stockings to prevent blood from pooling in the veins. This is especially useful in patients with varicose veins, which may pool a considerable volume of blood. A variety of such stockings are available, some ready-made, others made to order. The latter are more expensive but are also more effective and durable. Patients should put the stockings on in the morning before getting out of bed. Still another mechanical trick is to raise the head of the bed about 3 or 4 inches with wood blocks. This alters kidney function at night to cause increased salt retention.

If these countermeasures are not sufficient, the patient's physician may wish to try the drug fluorohydrocortisone. As the name implies, this drug is related to cortisone, the hormone of the adrenal cortex. Fluorohydrocortisone is a synthetic hormone that controls the metabolism of sodium chloride. It causes the kidney to retain more sodium chloride—and release less of it into the urine—than it would otherwise do. It is a very potent drug and has been helpful in the rare patient with severe low blood pressure complicating parkinsonism.

Midodrine is useful in Parkinson's disease patients with low blood pressure. This drug acts by stimulating the α-adrenergic receptors in the blood vessels, causing contraction, and thereby increasing pressure.

EFFECTS ON BLADDER AND BOWEL

Because the action of the bladder is under the influence of the sympathetic nerves, some weakening of bladder function is very occasionally experienced by patients when they first start levodopa treatment. The effect is relatively mild; indeed, much milder than the similar effect of the anticholinergic drugs. It is a relatively rare side effect of levodopa and seems to occur only in men. Rarely, patients report that they have more constipation on levodopa treatment, but there is no evidence that this is, in fact, a direct effect of the drug.

DISCOLORATION OF URINE AND SWEAT

A major portion of the levodopa absorbed by the intestine is removed from the circulation by the kidneys. The kidneys rapidly convert it to dopamine and then to a series of inactive substances. Some of these are pigments called *melanins*. They range in color from orange to red to brown and finally to black. The pigments are more likely to be formed if the urine is alkaline. Drops of urine reacting with alkaline materials, such as dried bleach in underclothing or bedsheets, may produce reddish or brownish stains. Many patients have been frightened by such stains, mistaking them for blood. Occasionally, patients note after passing urine that the water in the toilet bowl is tinged with red. This is especially likely to occur if the bowl was recently treated with some disinfectant solution. In case of doubt it is best of course to consult a physician. The urine can very quickly be examined to ascertain whether there has been bleeding into the urinary tract.

A very small amount of levodopa may also be secreted by the sweat glands. Rarely, some dark beads of sweat result and stain undergarments.

INTERACTIONS WITH OTHER DRUGS

Patients are often concerned that a drug prescribed by another doctor for some acute illness may interfere with their levodopa. For example, they may have been given an antibiotic to treat the flu or some other infection. Or a doctor may have prescribed an antihistamine to control some hay fever symptoms, or the dentist may want to administer Novocain before drilling. Many other examples come to mind. In nearly all these situations, there is no problem. Levodopa is a particularly forgiving drug and can be used with almost anything. Only a few interactions of any significance have been encountered.

The number one "no-no" is to combine a monoamine oxidase (MAO) inhibitor drug with levodopa. We have already explained the potentially dangerous interactions that can occur when levodopa and a MAO inhibitor are taken together. Under no circumstances should these agents be combined.

MAO inhibitor drugs had been tried in the treatment of parkinsonism before the introduction of levodopa but were soon abandoned as ineffective. They were tried again in combination with levodopa in the early days of experimentation with levodopa. The idea was to enhance and prolong the effect of levodopa. Although these drugs did enhance the effect of a given dose of levodopa, they did not prolong the duration of the response and, unfortunately, produced episodes of high blood pressure and very rapid pulse rates. The one exception is selegiline (Eldepryl).

Aside from this one serious interaction, there is little to fear. All that can happen is that the effect of levodopa may be diminished. The major tranquilizer drugs, which act by blocking the action of dopamine in the nervous system, simply diminish the actions of levodopa. Therefore, they should not be taken by patients on levodopa therapy. The drug metoclopramide (Reglan) employed to treat stomach disorders also blocks the action of dopamine and should be used cautiously if at all. Patients should also be cautious about taking vitamin preparations containing large amounts of vitamin B_6 (pyridoxine) because this vitamin can antagonize the effects of levodopa. The mechanism of this somewhat surprising interaction is explained in Chapter 10. Two calcium channel blockers (cinarrazine and flunarrazine) widely prescribed in Europe but not available in the United States may also block the effect of dopamine. Patients with Parkinson's disease should avoid these two drugs. Other calcium channel blockers used to treat heart conditions or high blood pressure may rarely worsen the symptoms of parkinsonism. Since this side effect is so infrequent, however, these drugs may be employed without undue worry in the vast majority of patients.

There is no problem in giving analgesics, antihistamines, vaccines, flu shots, or Novocain anesthesia to Parkinson's disease patients on levodopa treatment. Antibiotics sometimes cause diarrhea, thereby reducing the absorption of levodopa and temporarily worsening the symptoms of Parkinson's disease. Patients improve after the course of antibiotics is completed, and levodopa again is absorbed normally.

ENZYME INHIBITOR DRUGS

Carbidopa And Benserazide

The conversion of L-dopa to dopamine (see page 69) is controlled by a specific enzyme bearing the impressive scientific name l-aromatic amino acid decarboxylase. When discussing levodopa metabolism, we commonly refer to this enzyme by the short name *dopa decarboxylase*. Several drugs inhibit this enzyme and are therefore known to the pharmacologist as dopa decarboxylase inhibitors. A few of these inhibitors greatly increase the effect of a given dose of levodopa in Parkinson patients, and two of them are used in combination with levodopa: carbidopa and benserazide. The combination of carbidopa and levodopa in a single tablet is marketed under the trade name Sinemet. A similar combination containing levodopa and benserazide (marketed under the name *Madopar*) is not available in the United States. Each of these formulations is available in several strengths (see Appendix 1). In our experience these two preparations are very similar in their effect.

These drugs modify the body's metabolism of levodopa by inhibiting dopa decarboxylase and thus preventing the conversion of levodopa to dopamine. The key to their value in treating parkinsonism is that they are unable to enter the brain. The brain differs from all other organs in having the ability to regulate the admission of substances traveling through the body in the circulation. It has in effect a highly selective barrier. We call it the blood–brain barrier. It admits levodopa but not dopamine. Similarly, it does not admit carbidopa or benserazide. As a result of this curious circumstance, carbidopa and benserazide inhibit the conversion of levodopa to dopamine throughout the body *except* in the brain. Consequently, these agents greatly increase the proportion of levodopa taken by mouth that ultimately reaches the brain and is converted to dopamine. In effect, they protect the levodopa until it has a chance to reach the brain. The protection is not complete, but it is quite significant. In practice, approximately 80% less levodopa needs to be taken by mouth when the combination treatment is used than when levodopa is used alone. This means that a patient who needs 5 g of levodopa for symptom control now needs only 1 g. Instead of ten 0.5-g tablets of levodopa a day, an individual needs only four tablets of Sinemet or Madopar containing 0.25 g of levodopa each. Taking four small pills instead of ten large ones is a matter of some convenience. However, the major bonus of combining levodopa with a decarboxylase inhibitor is that it largely abolishes the action of levodopa on the vomiting center. The reason for this is that this area does not hide behind the blood–brain barrier. To do its work, the vomiting center must be able to sample the various substances traveling in the circulation. Thus carbidopa and benserazide gain access to the vomiting center and prevent the formation of dopamine there.

The practical consequences of this situation are considerable. First, a patient just starting levodopa therapy need not begin with very small doses and build up slowly over a period of months to the full dosage while waiting for the vomiting center to develop tolerance for levodopa. Instead many patients can reach full dosage within a matter of weeks if this is desired because of the severity of the symptoms. Second, the various precautions discussed earlier (see Nausea and Vomiting, below) to minimize levodopa-induced nausea and vomiting can now usually be ignored. Thus dose schedules can be set up in accord with the patient's need, without regard to mealtimes. The patient who requires levodopa immediately upon arising in the morning need not wait until after breakfast but can take the combination tablet even before getting out of bed. The patient who needs levodopa every 2 or 3 hours to maintain a smooth response throughout the day no longer needs to wait until the next meal but can take the combination tablet on an empty stomach. For these reasons, treatment with Sinemet or Madopar is much more convenient and agreeable to both patient and physician. Levodopa is now rarely used alone.

It must be admitted of course that all is not perfect even in the most perfect of all possible worlds. There are still patients, though very few, who feel some nausea despite taking levodopa in combination with carbidopa or benserazide. These few patients must heed the precautions (see Nausea and Vomiting, below) that were learned in the early days of levodopa therapy. One reason that the decarboxylase inhibitor may fail to protect all patients from activation of the vomiting center is that the amount of carbidopa in the lowest-strength Sinemet tablet may not be sufficient to prevent the formation of some dopamine in the vomiting center. The 10/100 Sinemet tablet contains 10 mg of carbidopa and 100 mg (or 0.10 g) of levodopa. The obvious solution to this is to take an additional amount of carbidopa separately. This is provided in the 25/100 Sinemet tablet containing 25 mg of carbidopa. Because this tablet is scored, it is possible to use a half tablet, that is, 12.5/50 mg, and still have enough carbidopa to prevent nausea. Since the introduction of the 25/100 tablet, nausea has been a rare occurrence. Those rare patients who still have nausea may be helped by using diphenidol (Vontrol) or trimethobenzamide (Tigan, Monarch Pharmaceuticals, Bristol, TN, U.S.A.).

If despite all these measures, nausea persists, one may have recourse to the drug domperidone (Motilium, Johnson & Johnson, New Brunswick, NJ, U.S.A.), which is routinely used in Europe and Canada to counter levodopa-induced nausea and stomach upsets. Unlike its close cousin metoclopramide (Reglan), it does not gain entry to the brain and thus does not risk blocking the desired effects of levodopa therapy on parkinsonism. Domperidone (AstraZeneca, Wilmington, DE, U.S.A.) is not available in the United States; it can be obtained from pharmacists in Europe, Canada, Mexico, and elsewhere. A 10-mg tablet taken with each dose of levodopa–carbidopa can effectively block the nausea. The daily medication schedule may need to be adjusted so that both drugs are taken together. Protection against the vomiting effect of levodopa is greater if the protecting drug is taken simultaneously with levodopa, before the nausea and vomiting begin. When the feeling of nausea has developed, it is too late to expect much benefit from the protecting drug.

Tolcapone and Entacapone

Another enzyme that controls the conversion of l-dopa to dopamine is cate-chol-O-methyl transferase (COMT). Entacapone (Comtan) and tolcapone (Tas-mar) are two newer drugs that block this conversion and therefore are known as COMT inhibitors. By slowing the conversion of l-dopa to dopamine in the blood, more l-dopa gets into the brain, where it is needed. These two drugs therefore enhance the beneficial effect of levodopa and in patients with fluctua-tions make the effectiveness of each dose last longer. These drugs must be used along with levodopa; they are ineffective if given alone. In a few patients, tol-capone has been associated with liver damage. All patients on this drug therefore must undergo periodic tests of liver function (a blood test).

Selegiline

We have already emphasized the dangers of taking a monoamine oxidase (MAO) inhibitor along with levodopa. The combination risks inducing attacks of high blood pressure (the "cheese reaction"). However, the drug selegiline (Elde-pryl)—a MAO inhibitor—is one very important exception to that warning; this drug is also known generically as deprenyl. Selegiline is an exception because there are two types of the enzyme MAO: type A, present in the adrenal glands, heart, liver, and other organs; and type B, present in the brain. Dopamine in the brain is metabolized mainly by MAO-B. Selegiline inhibits MAO-B, but not MAO-A, and thus can safely be taken with levodopa.

Taken in combination with levodopa–carbidopa (Sinemet) or levodopa–benserazide (Madopar), selegiline enhances the effects of levodopa, both the good and the side effects. The standard dosage is one 5-mg tablet twice daily, one after breakfast and one after lunch. Because of its resemblance to amphetamine and a slight amphetamine-like action that might cause insomnia, patients are usually advised not to take it later in the day. Patients under our care have taken it after dinner or even at bedtime, with no effect on their sleep. Some patients seem to respond as well to one tablet a day. Higher daily dosages are not recom-mended because, at dosages above 10 mg per day, the selectivity for MAO-B inhibition may be lost and MAO-A inhibition may begin to occur, bringing the risk of hypertensive reactions.

In practice, the effects of adding selegiline to a Sinemet or Madopar regimen seem about the same as the effects that could be expected from increasing the dosage of levodopa 20% to 25%. Dyskinesias may become more pronounced. It may then be necessary to reduce the dose of levodopa by about that proportion. Because selegiline inhibits the breakdown of dopamine by MAO-B, it prolongs somewhat the duration of the benefit yielded by each dose of levodopa. Thus it is useful in patients who experience a wearing off of levodopa between doses or on–off fluctuations. A moderate reduction in the fluctuations may be expected.

In our experience, it also improves the general quality of the response to levodopa treatment.

Selegiline seems to have few side effects of its own. The side effects are those of levodopa. Nausea is perhaps the most common side effect we have seen when adding selegiline to patients' Sinemet regimen. Usually, this occurs in patients who experienced nausea earlier with Sinemet alone and is easily controlled by reducing the dose to half a tablet a day for a few weeks and then gradually building up to the standard dosage of two tablets daily. Again, the use of antinausea drugs such as diphenidol (Vontrol) or trimethobenzamide (Tigan) has occasionally been necessary, but tolerance to selegiline has usually developed fairly rapidly, with nausea subsiding in a month or two.

In addition to enhancing the effects of levodopa, selegiline may lessen the symptoms of Parkinson's disease when given alone. In patients with newly diagnosed mild parkinsonism whose symptoms are bothersome but too minimal to require active treatment with levodopa, selegiline can delay the need for levodopa therapy for months to a year or more. Accordingly, it is often recommended as the initial treatment of newly diagnosed Parkinson's disease. Sinemet or a dopamine agonist is then added when needed in the usual manner. (See Chapter 9.) This delaying effect on the need for levodopa was thought several years ago to indicate that selegiline has a retarding effect on the progression of Parkinson's disease. But with further experience, most physicians have come to believe that selegiline itself helps the symptoms of early Parkinson's disease without slowing the disease process itself.

8

Imitators of Dopamine

No one who can remember what parkinsonism was like before levodopa can doubt that this drug brought a very great improvement over the drug treatments previously available. Great as this improvement was, however, levodopa was clearly not the final answer. From the earliest days of levodopa treatment, physicians have yearned for a still more effective drug. They have thought that some of the limitations of levodopa treatment stem from the fact that it has no effect itself but must first be converted to dopamine. For a number of theoretical reasons, it has seemed desirable to find a substance that would not need to be converted to the active agent but that could act like dopamine. Some of the side effects of levodopa then might not occur.

Many drugs directly imitating the action of dopamine have been tested in Parkinson's disease patients. Four of these—bromocriptine (Parlodel, Novartis Pharmaceuticals Corporation); pergolide (Permax, Athena Neurosciences, Inc., South San Francisco, CA, U.S.A.); pramipexole (Mirapex); and ropinirole (Requip)—are now regularly used in the treatment of parkinsonism. More are in various stages of development. These "imitators" of dopamine are properly termed *dopamine receptor agonists*. To understand the meaning of this term, it is necessary to think for a moment about how dopamine works in the nervous system.

We have described dopamine as a chemical messenger essential to the normal function of the brain. It is the means whereby the nerve cells of the substantia nigra communicate with the corpus striatum. These nerve cells form and store dopamine; they release it in the corpus striatum. The nerve cells of the striatum receive this messenger at special receptor sites on their surfaces that recognize and respond to dopamine but not to other naturally occurring chemical messengers. For example, the dopamine receptors will pay little attention to epinephrine, norepinephrine, serotonin, or other chemical messengers that are also normally present in the corpus striatum. They are highly specific for dopamine, and thus we may think of them as *dopamine receptors*.

Although the dopamine receptors are very selective regarding which chemical messengers they recognize, they can be fooled. Many substances are now known to act at the dopamine receptors in much the same way that dopamine does.

Drugs that can activate a receptor are known collectively as *agonists* of that receptor, in contrast to those drugs that can block the receptor and are thus termed *antagonists*.

The first dopamine receptor agonist to be tested in Parkinson patients was apomorphine. This drug has long been useful in medical practice as an emetic. It activates the dopamine receptors in the vomiting center and is used to induce vomiting. The late Dr. George Cotzias hypothesized that it might also act on the dopamine receptors in the corpus striatum and thereby control the symptoms of parkinsonism. In fact, earlier, in the 1950s, it was reported by Dr. Albert Schwab in Boston, that an injection of apomorphine temporarily reduced the tremor of Parkinson's disease. Dr. Cotzias gave apomorphine by mouth to a small number of patients in much the same way he had prescribed levodopa. That is, he started treatment with small doses that he gradually increased to allow his patients time to develop tolerance to the emetic action of apomorphine. With care and persistence, he was able to reach substantial doses, and these did in fact yield significant relief of the symptoms of parkinsonism. He estimated that apomorphine was 40% to 50% as effective as levodopa. However, the blood tests he carried out in his patients indicated that there was a toxic effect on the kidneys. Cotzias and his colleagues searched for other drugs that might have the same properties. They tested a synthetic agent similar to apomorphine, *N*-methyl aporphine. The results were similar.

Although this work failed to produce a new treatment, it did show that a dopamine receptor agonist could have a significant anti-Parkinson effect; it also gave impetus to the search for better and less toxic agonists. A totally different drug, piribedil (Trivastal), was also found, somewhat unexpectedly, to be a dopamine receptor agonist. It too was tested in Parkinson patients but was abandoned as relatively ineffective. Then a synthetic analogue of ergotamine, the alkaloid drug used in treating migraine, was found to be a powerful dopamine receptor agonist. This drug, bromocriptine (Parlodel), appeared to have some advantages over levodopa in animal experiments. For example, its action lasted for 5 to 6 hours, whereas levodopa acted for only 2 to 3 hours in the same animals. It was also much more potent. A very small dose seemed equal in effect to a very large dose of levodopa.

In 1973, Dr. Donald Calne and his colleagues in London tried bromocriptine for the first time in Parkinson patients. Definite effects were found with modest doses. Other investigators soon confirmed these results. After a decade of extensive experimental treatment at various doses, alone and in combination with other drugs, bromocriptine became established as a useful addition to levodopa.

This drug is about 50% as effective as levodopa in relieving the symptoms of parkinsonism. Although it can be used alone in some patients for a period of time, it is most useful when used in combination with levodopa. Unfortunately, it cannot fully substitute for levodopa. Probably the most important quality of this drug is that its action lasts longer than that of levodopa. It is thus most helpful in patients with the on–off effect who enjoy only a short-duration response from each dose of levodopa, even when taking it every 2 to 3 hours. Bromocriptine can reduce the fluctuations, making the "on" phases last longer and the "off" phases shorter and milder. It is especially useful for patients suffering painful muscle or "dystonic" cramps in their off phases.

The side effects are similar to those of levodopa. Loss of appetite, nausea, vomiting, lowering of blood pressure, involuntary movements, agitation, vivid dreams, nightmares, confusion, and hallucinations have all been reported. Tolerance to the nausea and vomiting takes place rapidly. Usually, only mild nausea is encountered, and it subsides within a matter of days. Loss of appetite also disappears quickly and may be replaced by an increase in appetite after a time. A few patients have complained of gaining weight, but this has been minimal. Rarely, blood pressure falls sufficiently to cause lightheadedness, dizziness, and faintness. It is also rare, but bromocriptine seems to activate long-quiescent peptic ulcer disease.

The major and most troublesome side effects have been mental disturbances. In the mildest cases the patient displays an unusual suspiciousness of loved ones and friends. This may be followed by anxiety, insomnia, and vivid dreams. If the drug is continued, episodes of confusion and visual hallucinations may develop. In the severest cases, the patient is irrational and agitated. The propensity of bromocriptine to induce these toxic mental effects is greater than that of levodopa or the anticholinergic drugs. Of course, as with similar side effects with other drugs, these undesired manifestations subside rapidly after the drug is stopped.

Despite its side effects and limitations, bromocriptine is a useful addition to the drugs now available to treat parkinsonism. It serves mainly as a supplement to levodopa. Used cautiously in specific situations, it can be very helpful. It is available in a 2.5-mg tablet and a 5-mg capsule. Although some benefit may be seen with doses of 2.5 to 5 mg three times daily, larger doses of 10 to 20 mg three times daily, or even more, may be needed to obtain a significant effect. Treatment is usually begun with one-half of a 2.5-mg tablet for 2 weeks to assure tolerance to the possible side effects. The dose is then increased to one-half tablet three times daily after meals; later, to a full tablet three times daily; and then to a 5-mg capsule three times daily. In this manner, the dose can slowly be increased as needed. We rarely exceed a daily total of 40 mg.

Small doses of bromocriptine added to levodopa have been found to improve the quality of the response to treatment in mild cases of parkinsonism not experiencing the on–off effect. Professor Rinne of Turku University in Finland treated a group of patients with both bromocriptine and levodopa from the outset of treatment. He found that patients on the combined treatment fared better than those on levodopa alone over the 5 years of the study. Many neurologists initiate treatment with bromocriptine early in the course of the disease when the first indications of cramps or fluctuations in the response to levodopa emerge.

Another dopamine receptor agonist, pergolide (Permax), was studied extensively in the early 1980s in many centers in the United States and finally approved for use in Parkinson's disease in 1989. It is more potent than bromocriptine and thus is used in smaller doses. The benefits and side effects of the two drugs are very similar. In animal experiments, the effects of pergolide last much longer than those of bromocriptine. One might thus expect that pergolide would be more helpful in patients with the on–off effect, but in clinical practice there is no clear difference between the two. When patients stop taking pergolide, the effects take 3 to 4 days to subside. It may then be necessary to increase the dose of levodopa to compensate for the loss of the beneficial effect of pergolide. Pergolide is available in 0.05-, 0.25- and 1.0-mg scored tablets, providing flexibility in adjusting the dosage. It is generally used in doses ranging from 0.25 to 2.0 mg three times daily.

Pramipexole (Mirapex) is one of the two newer dopamine agonists in general use for the past several years. It is generally taken three times per day, and the side effects and benefits are similar to those of other agonists. It comes in a number of tablet sizes, ranging from a low of 0.125 mg to a high of 1.5 mg. Pramipexole is usually started at 0.125 mg three times per day and increased slowly over many weeks and months. The generally effective dose range is between 2.5 and 3.5 mg per day but can be as high as 4.5 mg per day.

Ropinirole (Requip) is the most recent of the agonists to be approved by the FDA. It too is usually taken three times per day with benefits and side effects similar to those of the other agonists. It is manufactured in the widest dose range of all the agonists; the lowest-dose pill is 0.25 mg, and the highest dose is 5.0 mg. Ropinirole is started at 0.25 mg three times per day and increased slowly to as much as 24.0 mg per day. This is a large therapeutic range, and it may take many months for a patient to increase the dose into the effective range, which is between 9.0 and 15.0 mg per day. It is important for patients and families therefore to have patience and not give up before the dose is high enough to exert a beneficial effect.

Largely because of the work of Dr. Gerald Stern of the Middlesex Hospital, London, apomorphine has recently enjoyed renewed attention. Dr. Stern and his colleagues have developed its use in selected patients experiencing severe on–off fluctuations on levodopa therapy. The patients are trained to inject themselves with a solution of apomorphine when they are in an off state. A prompt response occurs, lasting about 45 minutes. The patients use syringes and needles similar to those used to administer insulin to diabetics. Dr. Stern places his patients on domperidone (Motilium) treatment to protect them from the nausea and vomiting that apomorphine might otherwise provoke. Some patients appear to benefit from this treatment. In our experience, however, only a few have found it worth the trouble and expense. The short duration of the response and the need to have the syringe and needle ready at the right moment limit its value. Apomorphine is not readily available in the United States.

More than 40 dopamine receptor agonists have been tested in clinical trials over the past 20 years. Most have been abandoned because of toxic side effects. They all appear to have about the same degree of efficacy and similar side effects. None has shown sufficient efficacy to be used as the initial or as the only drug in the treatment of parkinsonism. None quite equals the action of levodopa. The reason is still not clear. Experiments in animal models of parkinsonism suggest that some effect of levodopa other than the replenishment of brain dopamine stores may be important. We emphasized in Chapter 1 the depletion of dopamine in parkinsonism. There is also, however, a depletion of norepinephrine stores. Levodopa treatment may also, at least partially, correct the norepinephrine deficiency. The dopamine receptor agonists do not activate the brain norepinephrine receptors.

Another possible explanation for the limited effects of the dopamine receptor agonists studied to date may lie in the fact that there are at least two major types of dopamine receptors. These have been designated the D-1 and D-2 receptors on the basis of certain distinct chemical properties. Dopamine activates all these receptors. Bromocriptine activates only the D-2 receptor; it is actually an antagonist of the D-1 receptor! Pergolide is a weak D-1 and a strong D-2 receptor agonist. Several selective D-1 agonists are presently known, but they are unavailable for use in patients. Studies by various investigators of D-1 receptor agonists in animals indicated that normal bodily movement requires activation of both types of receptors. However, limited trials in patients have not shown benefit when these are used alone or in combination with levodopa. The question remains open whether action at the D-1 receptor will be helpful to Parkinson's disease patients.

9

Making Decisions About the Treatment of Early Parkinson's Disease

It is evident from the previous four chapters that many drugs are now available to treat Parkinson's disease. This chapter will provide basic information that every patient needs to know about the merits and controversies surrounding the different drug strategies as initial treatment in the early stages of disease. There is no single correct scheme of treatment that is best for all. Each person must discuss his or her specific situation with the treating physician and together come up with the best treatment regimen for that individual.

If we could slow down the progression of Parkinson's disease, there would be no question but to begin treatment with a neuroprotective agent (a drug that protects cells from dying). Unfortunately, no medications have been shown to slow the progression of Parkinson's disease. Our treatment aim therefore is primarily symptomatic, with the important secondary intention of minimizing the short- and long-term complications of Parkinson's disease. The two major motor complications of advanced Parkinson's disease are motor fluctuations (end-of-dose wearing off) and dyskinesias (involuntary abnormal movements). An unresolved controversy that is the major topic of this chapter concerns whether to start levodopa early or delay it, because levodopa may be implicated as a contributing factor to the onset of motor fluctuations and dyskinesias. Many patients state this problem by asking if they will become "immune" to levodopa or by saying that they have heard levodopa works for "only 5 years," after which it is ineffective. Neither of these statements is true, but it is a fact that as the years go by, increasing numbers of patients develop fluctuations and dyskinesias, making their anti-Parkinson control more erratic and difficult. It used to be said that after 5 years of treatment, up to 50% of patients had fluctuations and dyskinesias. A recent comprehensive study, however, detected only a 20% frequency of fluctuations 5 years after initiating treatment with levodopa in a large group of Parkinson's disease patients. This is still a large number but should remind us that not everyone will get these complications. We will review the evidence for and against the hypothesis that early levodopa treatment may contribute to the onset of motor fluctuations and dyskinesias.

It is currently thought that at least two major mechanisms are responsible for the occurrence of motor fluctuations and dyskinesias as Parkinson's disease advances: loss of brain dopamine storage capacity and change in dopamine receptor sensitivity.

Mechanism 1: loss of brain dopamine storage capacity. As Parkinson's disease progresses, dopamine-producing cells gradually decline. These cells not only produce dopamine but also store it, so that it can be released gradually to the dopamine receptors. It is important to remember that the cells store both the brain's own dopamine and the dopamine made from taking levodopa tablets. Early in the disease therefore, when there is a fair amount of reserve storage capacity for dopamine, the patient experiences a smooth response when he or she takes levodopa. As time progresses and the brain storage of dopamine decreases to a critically low level, the response to levodopa shortens and the patient experiences end-of-dose, wearing-off motor fluctuations. Whereas a tablet of levodopa previously lasted many hours or even days, it now produces a beneficial effect for only a few hours because not enough brain dopamine has been stored from each tablet to last for longer periods of time. It is thus hypothesized that as fewer and fewer cells remain to store dopamine, it becomes more likely that a patient will experience motor fluctuations. If levodopa increases the rate of cell loss and thereby decreases dopamine storage capacity, then it will increase the likelihood of hastening the onset of motor fluctuations.

Arguments suggesting that levodopa may increase the rate of dopamine cell loss are the following:

1. The metabolism of levodopa produces "free radicals," which are molecules that break down cell membranes and may cause increased cell death.
2. The brains of patients with Parkinson's disease have reduced ability to control "free radical" accumulation.
3. Drugs other than levodopa are not associated with the same degree of motor fluctuations as levodopa.
4. Patients taking levodopa get motor fluctuations.
5. When levodopa is added to a cell culture (in a test tube) of pure dopamine-producing cells, the rate of cell death is slightly increased.

Arguments suggesting that it is Parkinson's disease progression alone that is responsible for the rate of dopamine cell loss are the following:

1. There is no evidence for increased free radical damage in patients taking levodopa.
2. Studies using drugs that block free radical production (DATATOP) did not show a change in the progression of Parkinson's disease.

3. In the only clinical study to date aimed at determining if levodopa increases the progression rate of Parkinson's disease, Drs. Shirley Diamond and Charles Markham were unable to show that levodopa has any deleterious effect.
4. Drugs other than levodopa do not produce fluctuations to the same degree as levodopa simply because they do not have as powerful an anti-Parkinson effect.
5. Some patients get fluctuations almost immediately upon starting treatment, suggesting it is the disease rather than the drug that is the cause.
6. When levodopa is added to a cell culture of dopamine-producing cells and their supporting cells (the more normal situation in the brain), the rate of cell death is slightly decreased.

Mechanism 2: change in dopamine receptor sensitivity. As Parkinson's disease progresses, there is a gradual decline in dopamine-producing cells. These cells normally send messages (via dopamine) to the dopamine receptors. With dopamine loss, receptors do not receive an adequate number of messages and begin to behave abnormally, with increased sensitivity to the chemical messenger, dopamine. Early in the disease, when there is a fair amount of the brain's own dopamine, the patient experiences a smooth response with the addition of levodopa because the receptors are behaving normally. As time progresses, the concentrations of dopamine that used to provide a normal response now produce dyskinesias because the receptors are now behaving abnormally.

It is hypothesized that the manner in which levodopa is usually given may contribute to the abnormal sensitivity of the dopamine receptors with time. Generally, levodopa is given several times per day. In the earlier stages of disease, brain cells can store the excess dopamine provided by multiple doses of levodopa for use throughout the day. As the number of these cells and their capacity to store dopamine declines (see Mechanism 1), the dopamine receptors receive "pulses" of dopamine; that is, they begin to see larger, intermittent amounts of dopamine in the first couple of hours after each dose of levodopa, followed by a significant drop in dopamine levels until the next dose is taken by the patient and the cycle begins again. As the dopamine receptors see intermittent rather than smooth dopamine stimulation over the course of many years, they begin to react abnormally, and patients begin to experience intermittent dyskinesias and motor fluctuations.

Arguments suggesting that intermittent levodopa treatment may contribute to the onset of abnormal receptor sensitivity are the following:

1. Studies in Parkinson's disease patients show changes in receptor sensitivity with advancing disease and ongoing treatment.
2. Giving levodopa in a continuous, smooth fashion via a pump decreases fluctuations.
3. Studies in experimental animals show abnormal receptor sensitivity after long-term pulsed treatments with levodopa.
4. Other anti-Parkinson drugs are not as prone to produce dyskinesias as levodopa.

Arguments suggesting that intermittent levodopa treatment has little or nothing to do with the onset of abnormal receptor sensitivity are the following:

1. Abnormal receptor sensitivity simply may be related to disease progression and the gradual decline of brain dopamine.
2. Some patients begin to have dyskinesias very early in the course of treatment with levodopa.
3. Other anti-Parkinson drugs cannot be administered in large enough doses to produce dyskinesias because of unacceptable side effects.
4. A major study in which smoother dosing of levodopa was compared with more intermittent dosing did not show any difference in the incidence of fluctuations and dyskinesias between the two regimens.

It is important to note that the mechanisms and arguments outlined earlier are not proven. There are other reasons to explain the onset of fluctuations and dyskinesias that might come to light in the near future. One up-and-coming area of research is genetics. The human genome can be considered as the program that tells cells what to do. Such genetic programming may explain why some patients progress more rapidly than others, why only certain patients get motor fluctuations and dyskinesias, and why some patients get them earlier than others. It may have very little to do with treatment strategies. In the meantime, physicians try to use strategies based on these hypotheses together with the needs of each patient, aimed at minimizing fluctuations and perhaps even delaying their onset.

Based on the preceding discussion, there will be many appropriate strategies for starting treatment, almost as many as individual patients. We will therefore outline a number of possible approaches, although the following list is by no means comprehensive.

1. Delay the start of treatment until the patient finds that he or she cannot do something that is important to his or her social, psychological, or physical well-being. Almost everyone follows this approach, and the following discussion describes treatment strategies that may be used once a patient and physician have concluded that some form of treatment is necessary.
2. Begin with the lowest dose of levodopa (Sinemet) that improves the patient's symptoms.
3. Begin with a controlled-release form of levodopa (Sinemet CR).
4. Begin with a dopamine agonist such as bromocriptine (Parlodel), pergolide (Permax), pramipexole (Mirapex), or ropinirole (Requip).
5. Begin with one of a number of other drugs, such as selegiline (Eldepryl), amantadine (Symmetrel), or an anticholinergic (see Chapter 6).

If fluctuations start to appear once the patient is already on levodopa, a number of different approaches are available to help reduce this complication.

1. Give levodopa more frequently.
2. Switch to a controlled-release form of levodopa.

3. Add a catecho-O-methyl transferase (COMT) inhibitor such as tolcapone (Tasmar) or entacapone (Comtan).
4. Add a dopamine agonist.
5. Add one of a number of other drugs, such as selegiline, amantadine, or an anticholinergic.

We cannot overemphasize that there are no definitely right or wrong strategies. Remember, every patient is different, with different needs and different sets of problems. Patients and family members should discuss their fears and needs with their doctor and come up with a set of strategies that are acceptable to everyone. At the time we are writing this book, a research study is in progress to determine whether delaying the use of levodopa delays the onset of fluctuations and dyskinesias. This study by the Parkinson Study Group and supported by the National Institutes of Health, called the ELLDOPA study, is being carried out under the direction of Dr. Ira Shoulson of the University of Rochester and Dr. Stanley Fahn of Columbia University. Patients should ask their physicians whether or not the study has been completed and what the results are.

10

Special Remedies for Special Symptoms

In the preceding chapters, we described the major anti-Parkinson drugs: levodopa, the dopamine-receptor agonists, selegiline (Eldepryl), the catechol-O-methyl transferase (COMT) inhibitors, amantadine, and the anticholinergics. In general, these drugs relieve all or at least some symptoms related to the classic triad: tremor, rigidity, and bradykinesia. There remains a miscellaneous group of drugs whose acquaintance many patients are apt to make sooner or later. They are not specific for parkinsonian symptoms but are used to treat symptoms that are very common, such as insomnia, anxiety, and constipation. Some discussion of these drugs is appropriate because Parkinson's disease patients may react differently to these commonly used agents, and some of these drugs may interact adversely with the major anti-Parkinson drugs. We have already discussed some of these less classic symptoms of Parkinson's disease in Chapter 4. This chapter will expand on that material with more specific references to available treatments.

POSTURAL AND ACTION TREMOR (PROPRANOLOL)

The drug propranolol (Inderal, Wyeth–Ayerst Laboratories, Philadelphia, PA, U.S.A.) is used mainly to treat irregularity of the pulse and, to a lesser extent, to control high blood pressure. It may be used for these purposes in Parkinson patients with heart disease, irregular heart rate, or high blood pressure. It may also be used to protect the heart from the possibility of levodopa causing palpitations or episodes of abnormal heart rhythm in patients who are subject to palpitations.

Propranolol, however, has also been used occasionally because it seems to have a favorable effect on tremor, at least in some patients. Because the drug has an important action on the heart, it must be used with care. It is not recommended for patients who have asthma or have had heart failure, since it may exacerbate these conditions.

Very occasionally, a patient who still has some disturbing tremor despite good control of other symptoms of Parkinson's disease may enjoy a good response to this drug. Unfortunately, propranolol has no effect on other symptoms.

Propranolol is commonly used to treat the symptom of tremor in the condition known as *benign essential tremor* or *familial tremor* (see Chapter 3). This is sometimes confused with parkinsonism because the tremor often bears a superficial resemblance. However, none of the other manifestations of Parkinson's disease develop in persons with essential or familial tremor, even after 40 to 50 years. On closer examination, their tremor differs in a number of respects from that of Parkinson's disease. One of these differences is that the tremor is not present at rest; instead, it is present during movement or on maintaining a posture for a moment. Thus it is an action and a postural tremor. Another difference is that in essential tremor, the head and the voice are commonly involved; this rarely, if ever, occurs in Parkinson's disease. Finally, essential tremor responds differently to various drugs. In particular, it can be suppressed for a few hours by alcohol, whereas the tremor of Parkinson's disease is not reduced as significantly by alcohol. A highball or a glass of sherry dramatically diminishes the former for a few hours but not the latter. The various minor tranquilizers may also effectively reduce essential tremor, paralleling the action of alcohol. Levodopa has no effect on essential tremor but can greatly reduce or abolish the tremor of Parkinson's disease.

Several new drugs, closely related to propranolol, are available. One of these, metoprolol (Lopressor), is used primarily in treating high blood pressure. It is not as effective as propranolol against tremor but has much less risk of exacerbating asthma.

MINOR TRANQUILIZERS AND HYPNOTICS

Minor tranquilizers are sometimes prescribed for patients with tremor persisting despite treatment with the usual anti-Parkinson drugs. They may also be given to relieve the sense of inner restlessness and nervousness that may occur as a symptom of Parkinson's disease or as a side effect of anti-Parkinson drugs. These symptoms most frequently occur when the effect of levodopa wears off between doses. It is better to deal with them by adjusting the doses or the schedule, or switching to a slow-release formulation, than to use tranquilizers. However, in some instances, the mild tranquilizers may be helpful. Those most commonly used are lorazepam (Ativan, Wyeth–Ayerst Laboratories), diazepam (Valium, Roche Products), oxazepam (Serax, Wyeth–Ayerst Laboratories), and alprazolam (Xanax, Pharmacia and Upjohn Company). These drugs are called "minor" tranquilizers to distinguish them from the "major" tranquilizers, such as chlorpromazine (Thorazine), trifluoperazine (Stelazine), and haloperidol (Haldol), which are used primarily in psychiatric practice to treat severe mental illness. The major tranquilizers block the action of dopamine in the brain and consequently can cause parkinsonism. They therefore should not normally be given to Parkinson patients. The minor tranquilizers are entirely different and do not cause parkinsonism. They may, in fact, be quite useful but should be used sparingly and only as needed.

The minor tranquilizers can cause drowsiness, incoordination, dizziness, and confusion, and occasionally seem to increase the bradykinesia, or slowness of movement, of Parkinson's disease. Moreover, some persons may become psychologically dependent on or habituated to these drugs. Patients who use these drugs heavily for a period of time and then suddenly stop taking them may suffer withdrawal symptoms, including nervousness, agitation, and even (rarely) convulsions. However, we have never encountered a Parkinson patient who became dependent on these drugs, perhaps because we are careful to prescribe them sparingly.

SLEEPLESSNESS

What can the Parkinson patient with insomnia take to induce sleep? Preferably, of course, nothing. If levodopa (whether used alone or in a combined formulation with carbidopa or benserazide) seems responsible for insomnia, the bedtime dose should be avoided; if the drug is necessary, it might be reduced 50%. The presence of frequent nightmares may be a sign that levodopa is responsible for insomnia. Several old, nonmedical tricks may be quite helpful in inducing sleep at night, including a warm drink (e.g., a glass of warm milk) or even a brandy at bedtime. If insomnia is still a problem, a mild sedative such as chloral hydrate may be used. This is a very old and mild, short-acting sedative that leaves no hangover and is least apt of all the available hypnotics to cause confusion. It is made in the form of 250- and 500-mg capsules. Usually, one 500-mg capsule on retiring is successful, but another capsule may be taken an hour later if necessary. Two capsules (1.0 g) may be used on retiring if one is not effective. A mild tranquilizer such as lorazepam, 1 mg at bedtime, may also be helpful.

Parkinson patients more commonly have no trouble falling asleep on initially retiring. Rather their problem is that they wake up after several hours and then cannot get to sleep again. If there are recurrent Parkinson symptoms at that time—stiffness, cramps, or just slowness—and the patient cannot find a comfortable position, then an additional dose of levodopa–carbidopa (Sinemet) or levodopa–benserazide (Madopar) may be helpful. Using a slow-release preparation such as Sinemet CR or Madopar HBS at bedtime will often provide an extra hour or two of sleep by delaying the wearing off that causes the patient to wake up.

Sometimes multiple awakenings during the night or early morning awakening is a sign of depression (also see Chapter 4). Standard antidepressants such as the serotonin reuptake inhibitors (e.g., paroxetine and sertraline) or the tricyclic antidepressants (e.g., nortriptyline, amitriptyline, and imipramine) may be helpful in reducing insomnia in such cases. It is important to recall that these drugs are not sleeping medications and therefore do not work immediately. With many of these drugs, the dose must be increased gradually and the beneficial effect is not seen for 6 to 8 weeks after the therapeutic dose is achieved. Furthermore, these drugs must be continued daily to maintain good sleep. They cannot be taken as needed. Many patients who are not depressed also are helped by these drugs, presumably because they normalize the abnormal sleep–wake cycle in patients with Parkinson's disease.

Parkinson patients should avoid over-the-counter sedatives such as Compoz (Medtech, Inc.), Sominex (GlaxoSmithKline), Sleep-eze (Christine Columbus, Inc.), Nytol (Block Drug Company), and others. These preparations all contain scopolamine (hyoscine) as an active ingredient, in quantities comparable to those formerly employed in treating parkinsonism. (See the discussion of solanaceous alkaloids in Chapter 6.) They also contain an over-the-counter antihistamine, methapyrilene hydrochloride, which, like other antihistamines, also has some anticholinergic activity. The addition of these agents to a Parkinson patient's existing drug regimen, which may already include some anticholinergic agents, may carry the patient over the threshold of anticholinergic toxicity. Consequently, Parkinson patients are less able to tolerate the side effects commonly produced by these medications. On the other hand, the anticholinergic properties of these formulations may have some beneficial effect on the symptoms of parkinsonism. Patients should consult their doctors before trying them, however, to minimize the chance of an unpleasant interaction with their own anti-Parkinson drug treatment.

TREATMENT OF HALLUCINATIONS AND PARANOIA

Since the advent of levodopa therapy, most patients with Parkinson's disease are living longer. Consequently, more are encountering some of the complications of advancing disease. Dr. Christopher Goetz and his colleagues at Rush–Presbyterian–St. Luke's Medical Center in Chicago have emphasized that the presence of hallucinations or paranoia is the single most important factor determining whether a Parkinson patient will need long-term nursing home care. It is therefore important to keep these symptoms controlled. As discussed in Chapter 7, levodopa can sometimes provoke hallucinations or paranoia. The other drugs used to treat parkinsonism in conjunction with levodopa, however, are even more prone to exacerbate these mental aberrations.

Many steps taken to reduce hallucinations and paranoia inevitably worsen the motor symptoms of Parkinson's disease. Initially, decreasing the secondary drugs may control hallucinations and paranoia. Selegiline. anticholinergic drugs, and dopamine-receptor agonists are discontinued one at a time. Most patients and spouses willingly trade lessened psychotic behavior for more tremor or slowness. Sometimes small doses of the major tranquilizers discussed in the previous section can reduce hallucinations or paranoia; these drugs are rarely helpful for very long and can exacerbate the parkinsonism. Over the past several years, Dr. Joseph Friedman at Brown University and others have advocated the use of clozapine (Clozaril) to treat psychosis associated with parkinsonism. This drug blocks the effect of dopamine mostly in the limbic system and cortex (the part of the brain responsible for hallucinations) and has less effect on dopamine in the corpus striatum. It therefore does not worsen the symptoms of Parkinson's disease. Unfortunately, clozapine can be dangerous, since it may depress neutrophils (white blood cells) to critical levels. All patients on clozapine are required to undergo weekly blood tests, and the drug must be stopped if the number of neutrophils drops below the danger point.

DIURETICS (LEG SWELLING)

Swelling of the feet due to the accumulation of water in the tissues (edema) of the legs and feet is a common manifestation of parkinsonism (also see Chapter 4). It is often more marked in one leg, nearly always the leg on the side where the first symptoms occurred. The causes of this swelling are not fully understood. One reason may be that there is less muscular activity in that limb due to the bradykinesia of parkinsonism. It is wise to try simple symptomatic treatments first. These include increased walking, elastic stockings, and elevation of the feet when sitting for long periods of time. If these measures fail, the swelling can be diminished by diuretic agents (i.e., drugs that increase the volume of urine passed in a day). Milder diuretics such as hydrochlorothiazide (Hydrodiuril, Merck & Co. Inc.) may effectively relieve this swelling. Usually, only one dose once or twice a week is necessary. The drug should be taken only with a doctor's prescription.

If the swelling was induced by the drug amantadine (Symmetrel), it should subside when that drug is stopped, although it may require several weeks to disappear. The doctor may advise further treatment.

LAXATIVES (CONSTIPATION)

Chronic constipation is a familiar symptom of Parkinson's disease (also see Chapter 4). It results from a general slowing of the muscular action of the bowel or of muscular action in other organs. As mentioned earlier, constipation is also often exacerbated by the drugs used in treating parkinsonism. The tendency of Parkinson patients to drink little water is a further complicating factor. Consequently, many patients need to take laxatives.

We urge patients to try natural means of maintaining normal bowel habits. This means making an effort to drink more water, to eat adequate roughage and high-fiber foods; and to ingest prunes, prune juice, or figs regularly. A favorite regimen is stewed prunes, bran cereal, and apple sauce for breakfast. Patients must not eat bananas, since they increase constipation. Failing all this, one must resort to laxatives. Several classes of laxatives must be considered.

First, there are bulk laxatives that work by retaining water in the stools. Patients who pass small, hard stools—really dehydrated stools—may benefit from this measure alone. A common laxative in this class is Metamucil (Proctor & Gamble, Cincinnati, OH, U.S.A.), available over the counter. A tablespoonful stirred in one glass of water a day may suffice.

Another useful preparation is the fecal softener dioctyl sodium sulfosuccinate (also known as docusate sodium). A great many proprietary over-the-counter preparations containing this ingredient are available. One capsule one, two, or three times daily may be used. Generally, these are used on a regular daily maintenance basis by Parkinson patients.

If these measures are inadequate, an "irritant" laxative that stimulates the bowel directly may be required. Milder ones such as bisacodyl (Dulcolax, Novartis Consumer) are preferable. Some preparations combine such a stimulant with the fecal softeners mentioned earlier. The pharmacist can give advice about a suitable one, or the patient can check the label on the packages on the supermarket shelf, looking for the two ingredients dioctyl sodium sulfosuccinate (docusate sodium) and bisacodyl. We have also found lactulose helpful in some cases of severe constipation. We have found that cisapride (Propulsid, Jansen Pharmaceutica Inc., Titusville, NJ, U.S.A.) may also alleviate constipation in many patients with Parkinson's disease without causing undue side effects such as diarrhea. This drug increases the movement of stool through the colon by stimulating the nerves to the intestine. A physician must prescribe it.

Finally, many patients have a laxative habit acquired long before Parkinson's disease developed. They may prefer to continue using their old favorites. As a last resort, enemas may be required to maintain adequate evacuation.

ARTIFICIAL TEARS

The reduced frequency of spontaneous eye blink that is common in parkinsonism may result in some redness and dryness of the eyes and eyelids. (See Chapter 4 for other visual complaints.) The lids may become encrusted. Patients feel some irritation, a dry, burning feeling in the eyes. Usually, the major anti-Parkinson drugs restore eye blink to more normal frequency; with improvement in the normal "windshield wiper" function of the eyelids, these symptoms are relieved. However, if there is still some eye discomfort, irrigating the eyes with artificial tear solutions may be helpful. Various preparations of artificial tears can be purchased at local drug stores over the counter. They reproduce the salt concentration of natural tears. If symptoms are not relieved by this simple measure, medical advice should be sought.

TREATMENT FOR SEBORRHEA

The increased activity of the sebaceous glands of the skin in patients with Parkinson's disease commonly results in a somewhat greasy appearance of the face and forehead (seborrhea); occasionally, some patients have irritation and inflammation of the skin (seborrheic dermatitis). The seborrhea and the secondary dermatitis are reduced by treatment, especially by levodopa, and are rarely serious problems. To prevent the irritation, the oily secretion should be removed daily by washing the affected areas with a bland or neutral soap, with gentle scrubbing using an abrasive sponge or a face cloth. A commonly used soap formulation is the acne aid bar available at most drug stores. Dermatitis responds to a variety of lotions containing small amounts of hydrocortisone or related agents, but these require a doctor's prescription. Lotions, however, will seal in the irritating oily secretions of the skin, and so they should be applied after washing or scrubbing the affected areas.

A variety of hair lotions are available over the counter that may satisfactorily control excessive dandruff. One of the more effective contains selenium and is marketed under the name Selsun. A more concentrated solution of selenium is also available with a doctor's prescription. Many authorities advise that selenium preparations be used sparingly because they may cause hair loss if used excessively. It is best to reserve them as a last resort and then use them only occasionally.

DRUGS FOR LEG CRAMPS

Foot and leg cramps are a bona fide Parkinson's disease symptom, although rarely the initial symptom of the disease. They are most often due to wearing off of the levodopa benefit. Typically, they occur early in the morning when patients first get out of bed, but may also occur, or recur, during the day as the "dopa effect" wears off between doses. This "end-of-dose" dystonia is associated with spasm of the muscles of the calf and sole of the foot, in-turning of the foot, and clawing of the toes. Measures to counteract motor fluctuations generally alleviate or prevent these cramps. These include giving additional doses of levodopa/carbidopa (Sinemet) or levodopa–benserazide (Madopar), changing to a slow-release formulation (Sinemet CR; Madopar HBS), or adding a secondary anti-Parkinson drug. The dopamine-receptor agonists—bromocriptine (Parlodel), pergolide (Permax), pramipexole (Mirapex), and ropinirole (Requip)—are the most effective in combating these cramps. One may also try lioresal (Baclofen, Watson Laboratories, Inc., Corona, CA, U.S.A.) at the recommended dosage of 10 mg three times daily. Double this amount, however, may be needed to yield substantial relief. Some individuals have difficulty tolerating these doses of baclofen owing to nausea, dizziness, and drowsiness. Some physicians have recommended vitamin E (α-tocopherol) to prevent nocturnal cramps, but it has not been effective in our patients.

TRICKS TO HELP FREEZING

When freezing occurs and the feet feel glued to the floor (see Chapter 4 for more details), the patient should practice rocking from side to side, swinging the arms, and counting a marching cadence out loud. If this fails to get the patient moving, he or she should think about something else and try again. There are many tricks to help break through the "block," but not all of them work for every individual. Patients may try marching in place for a few steps, gently touching the "frozen" leg with the hand, stepping over an inverted cane, stepping over a partner's foot, or using a walker or shopping cart, just to name a few of the more common tricks to help freezing.

TIPS FOR PROBLEM SITUATIONS

Patients having particular trouble with their equilibrium during walking should have more formal gait-training exercises under the supervision of a physical therapist, preferably in a properly equipped physical medicine facility. Several suggestions have often proved helpful. First, consider shoes. If the patient shuffles, he or she will probably do better in shoes with leather or hard-composition soles. Shoes with rubber soles, especially crepe rubber, may be more comfortable to wear but cannot easily slide on most surfaces. Consequently, shuffling with a soft rubber sole is likely to make the foot stick to one spot, possibly causing loss of balance and a fall.

Patients who tend to step backward a few steps involuntarily (retropulsion)—and are thus subject to falling backward—may benefit from wearing shoes with heels. A heel lift inside the shoe may also help. Slippers with flat heels or no heels tend to increase the tendency to retropulsion. On the other hand, patients who have more difficulty with propulsion (falling forward) may do better on low or flat heels. Scatter rugs and mats are an additional hazard for patients who shuffle. It may be a wise precaution to remove them from the home. Doorsills may also be a problem, since freezing and festination indoors occur particularly at doorways. If necessary, a carpenter can easily be remove doorsills.

Patients who have trouble getting out of chairs should learn to avoid deep, upholstered chairs, especially those with low seats and soft cushions. They should try to choose instead straight-backed wooden chairs, preferably with arm rests, such as the traditional "captain's chair." The exercise described earlier can be used to get out of chairs. The patient should be sure to move forward to the edge of the seat, position the feet for proper leverage, and push up with both hands, leaning forward while getting up. If the patient needs help getting up from a chair, merely holding his or her hand and providing slight support may suffice. The mere contact of the hand seems to provide a necessary reference point. The sensation seems more important than the actual force or support provided. If that does not do the trick, the patient's companion may then place one hand on the patient's head and push forward gently but firmly. As the patient then tries again to get up, he or she may exert considerable back pressure against the companion's hand; however, the patient nearly always can rise briskly. Very little pressure is usually required. One can often help patients who have great difficulty in getting up with the pressure of one finger. It is much easier to help them in this way than to stand in front and pull up and forward with the hands. That may sometimes be needed, but one must be careful. Patients can be pulled up to standing only to fall on top of their helpers, with both ending up on the floor.

Reclining chairs can be obtained with a spring-loaded, lever-actuated, or motor-driven seat that pushes the patient up and forward on arising. Some patients find these chairs very helpful, but those with poor equilibrium may have difficulty. As they are pushed up and forward, they must be able to step forward. Patients who have difficulty standing and stepping forward may instead fall forward. We strongly advise a patient contemplating the purchase of such a chair to try it out first and be sure that it is actually helpful.

A simpler trick is to have the rear legs of the patient's favorite chair raised about 2 inches (5 or 6 cm) with blocks or a crossbeam. This gives the seat a slight forward tilt that makes it easier for the patient to get up yet does not make the chair less comfortable.

A cane provides less support to the Parkinson patient with a walking problem than might be expected. Even walkers are often disappointing. The patient with poor balance and subject to episodes of retropulsion simply falls backward—cane, walker, and all. Canes can be helpful to the patient with propulsion, and many patients do learn to use them effectively. Four-legged canes are helpful to patients with poor equilibrium. There are many varieties of canes and walking aids, and the patient should be trained in their proper use by a physical therapist. The therapist can also ascertain what type of device will be most helpful. Many patients use the cane not for support but as a guide, placing it on the floor slightly ahead of the foot about to step forward. This tells the brain where to put the foot down for the next step. It provides "sensory reinforcement," just as counting a cadence or walking over markers on the floor does.

Patients with severely impaired walking and poor equilibrium who are subject to frequent falls may, nevertheless, have very good stepping movements; they may be able to walk well, providing they are accompanied by someone who can catch them in time to prevent a fall. Such patients should have a brief daily walk with someone in attendance as a form of exercise.

Attention to the disposition of furniture around the house helps prevent injuries in case of falls. There should be an adequate rail on stairways. Hand bars on the wall near the bathtub and toilet should be installed. The toilet seat can be raised an inch or two with blocks. A chair can be placed in the shower stall or in the bathtub to render bathing easier and safer. Rubber bath mats should help reduce the chance of falls in the bathroom.

Those patients who have difficulty dressing, buttoning clothes, tying shoes, and so on because of lack of fine control of finger movements may benefit from several modifications of their clothing. Where possible, zippers or patches of adhesive cloth can be used instead of buttons. Polo shirts or T-shirts may be used in place of front-buttoned shirts. Shoelaces may be replaced by elastic laces that do not need to be tied or untied. Loafers or similar slip-on shoes without laces may be even more comfortable.

SPEECH EXERCISES

Patients whose speech is difficult for others to understand may benefit from practicing singing and reading aloud. Read the headlines from the daily newspaper, exaggerating the enunciation of each syllable. Sit before a mirror and watch the movements of the lips and tongue while reciting. Go slowly, breathe deeply, and forcefully blow out each syllable separately and loudly to practice projecting the voice. Listen carefully for each consonant and pause between the words. Recite to a measured beat marked by your hand or foot.

Patients are often not fully aware of their speech impairments. There seems to be some defect in their auditory self-monitoring. It may thus help to practice speaking into a tape recorder. Listen as you play back the phrase or newspaper headline you have just recited. Do it again, trying to correct the deficiencies you heard. By repeating this several times at one sitting, you will find that it is possible to improve speech function to a considerable degree.

If speech impairment is a major problem, ask your doctor to refer you to a qualified speech therapist.

CHEWING AND SWALLOWING

Making faces before a mirror helps to maintain the mobility of the facial muscles. Grin, frown, smile, snarl, pout, whistle, and puff out the cheeks.

If chewing and swallowing food is a problem, make an effort to chew first on one side, then on the other. Note the sound of the teeth while chewing; maintain the rhythm. Swallow small, well-chewed morsels only. Avoid the common habit of quickly swallowing half-chewed food.

SENSORY REINFORCEMENT

In the exercises we have discussed, we have stressed the importance of sensory stimuli. Counting a marching cadence out loud, using visual cues to guide the feet, and rocking from side to side to provoke stepping are all means of enhancing the sensory stimuli with which we normally, although unconsciously, monitor motor performance in complex activities. Consciously adding strong stimuli addressed to sight, hearing, and the sense of the body's position in space serves to reinforce the normal physiologic mechanisms underlying the performance of complex motor acts such as walking, talking, getting out of a chair, and so on. This sensory reinforcement is a useful principle in physical therapy, especially in the therapy of Parkinson patients. Patients can learn to make effective use of it in many circumstances, in their own way. Many of our patients have discovered this principle by themselves. One controlled his drooling tendency by constantly keeping a piece of raw carrot in his mouth. Its mere presence served to stimulate an increased frequency of swallowing and thus prevented the excessive accumulation of saliva in the mouth. Another had nails placed in the heels of her shoes. She listened to the resulting "click clack" as she walked. She found that it made her conscious of the rhythm of her walking and prevented episodes of festination that had been troubling her gait. Many patients have discovered other similar tricks that have helped them function better.

The principle of sensory reinforcement is employed in the formal physical therapy of Parkinson patients with good effect. Walking exercises, for example, are done in a group session with a number of patients to the beat of a drum. Calisthenics are similarly done in a group to the accompaniment of music with a strong rhythmic beat.

CHRONIC CARE FACILITIES

Ultimately, the patient with far-advanced Parkinson's disease may become too great a burden for the family, and at that point placement in a nursing home or chronic care hospital must be considered. Each case of course is different and must be evaluated on its individual merits. Some families are able to set up what is in effect a nursing home at home, with hospital equipment, private nurses and attendants, and so on. Most families, however, lack the resources—personal, emotional, and financial—to pursue such a demanding course. Moreover, it is not necessarily the best course for the patient. It is rarely possible to reproduce at home all the services and quality of care that are provided by the better nursing homes. For many patients rendered invalid by severe parkinsonism, a nursing home is preferable. Before making the final decision to seek nursing home placement, the patient and family will probably meet with a medical social worker.

Contact with a medical social worker first may be made in the hospital at the request of the patient's doctor. It may be arranged while the patient is at home through the visiting nurse service. The social worker here provides an essential service. The worker can review with the patient, the spouse, or other relative assuming responsibility for the patient's needs the available resources, doctor's recommendations, and prognosis. Applications to suitable homes can then be initiated. The spouse or other responsible person should, if possible, visit the various facilities being considered. In most areas there is a substantial waiting period for admission to a chronic care facility. It may be 2 to 3 months or more before a vacancy is likely to open up in a desirable home. Thus the patient may have to go home for a time to await admission to the nursing home of his or her choice.

Among the things to consider in choosing a nursing home is proximity to family members. It is very important that they find it easy to visit patients as often as possible. This ensures both better nursing home care and a psychological lift for the patient. A second consideration is the availability of good physical therapy. Is there a suitably equipped physical therapy facility? Are full-time physical therapists employed? Can bedside therapy be given if needed? In even the patient with the most far-advanced case of Parkinson's disease who is confined to bed and chair, physical therapy can offer much relief of discomfort and help with specific troublesome symptoms. Active and passive movement of the limbs, training in the fine art of using a wheelchair to full advantage, and ambulating with support if necessary can all make significant contributions to the patient's comfort and general well-being at this stage of the disease. It goes almost without saying that friendly and cooperative nursing and ancillary staff is important. Those in charge should be open to suggestions from patients and family members.

11

Surgical Treatment of Parkinsonism

HISTORICAL PERSPECTIVE

The surgical treatment of Parkinson's disease received a lot of attention in the 1950s and the 1960s. A variety of surgical procedures were rapidly developed during those years at medical centers throughout the world. With the advent of levodopa during the years from 1968 to 1970, the surgical treatment of parkinsonism was suddenly largely abandoned. The benefits of levodopa treatment were so remarkable in comparison with the effects achieved with our best previous medical treatment that surgery was reserved only for those patients who tolerated levodopa poorly or had persistent tremor despite optimal drug treatment. As a result, the number of operations performed fell sharply, and many surgeons stopped performing the procedure altogether.

A few neurologists and neurosurgeons, however, continued to offer the procedure and gradually improved the techniques. New imaging methods, such as computerized x-ray tomography (called the CAT or CT scan) and magnetic resonance imaging (MRI), developed in the 1980s, and computers capable of rapidly carrying out the necessary geometric calculations have made a surgical technique called *stereotactic surgery* simpler and more precise. Recently, better understanding of the basal ganglia and the effects of precisely placed lesions in the brain have sparked a renewed interest in brain surgery for parkinsonism. Although it is in no sense a cure and is useful in only a relatively small number of patients, modern brain surgery has a definite, if limited, place in the treatment of parkinsonism.

The first surgical efforts to alleviate parkinsonism were made during the 1930s. Various destructive operations were carried out in which some region of the cerebral cortex was removed or fibers deep in the brain were cut. The idea, stated somewhat crudely, was simply to damage the motor pathways enough to diminish tremor and rigidity without causing appreciable weakness. The results were mediocre and unpredictable, and the operations were relatively hazardous. Better procedures gradually evolved, largely from thoughtful trial and error and astute observation of accidental results. Dr. Russell Myers, a neurosurgeon then working at the Long Island College Hospital in New York, made an interesting discovery in 1939 while operating on a Parkinson patient with a brain tumor. When he cut through a part of the corpus striatum, tremor and rigidity on the opposite side of the body suddenly diminished. Taking advantage of this chance observation, he repeated the procedure in several more Parkinson patients. After trying a number of modifications based on the knowledge of brain anatomy available at the time, he found that the best effect could be achieved by severing a very small bundle of nerve fibers, deep in the brain, called the *ansa lenticularis*. This bundle could be severed without producing any apparent ill effect, and the result was an appreciable reduction of tremor and rigidity in some patients. It was, however, very difficult to reach a small fiber bundle deep in the brain with a scalpel, without inflicting damage upon other brain structures. Complications were serious and frequent, and few operations were actually done.

Many surgeons around the world tried to solve the problem of cutting that small fiber bundle safely and effectively. The most successful procedure turned out to involve a technique known as *stereotactic surgery*. The technique had long been employed in experimental brain surgery in animals. Drs. Henry T. Wycis and Ernest Spiegel, working at Temple University Hospital in Philadelphia, and Dr. Hiro Narabayashi, working independently in Tokyo, adapted this technique to human patients in 1948. They lowered a long needlelike probe into the brain through a small burr hole in the overlying skull. The direction and depth of the needle were carefully calculated from landmarks located on x-ray films of the patient's head. Placing the probe in the desired place was a simple problem in spatial or three-dimensional geometry, and it could be done with considerable precision. When the probe was positioned satisfactorily, a solution of alcohol could be injected or an electrical current run from its tip, thereby destroying a small amount of brain tissue and severing the nerve fiber bundle. Drs. Wycis and Spiegel called their operation *ansotomy*.

That small nerve fiber bundle identified as the target by Dr. Myers back in 1939 connects a structure called the *globus pallidum* (from the Latin, meaning "pale body") to another called the *thalamus*. Some surgeons chose the pallidum as their target. The operation was called *pallidotomy*. Others chose the termination of those fibers in the thalamus, calling their operation *thalamotomy*. Similar results were obtained using all three procedures. With the technology available in the 1960s, it was easier to locate the thalamus, and the results appeared to be better and the side effects less frequent and less severe than those with pallidotomy. Thus thalamotomy became the standard stereotactic operation for parkinsonism.

Various techniques of stereotactic surgery were developed. One that received much publicity was the cryosurgical technique developed by the late Dr. Irving Cooper at St. Barnabas Hospital in New York in the 1960s. Dr. Cooper used a needle with a system of tiny tubes through which a refrigerant solution of liquid nitrogen could be pumped. The effect was to freeze a small area of brain. Most stereotactic surgeons, however, used a radiofrequency current delivered from the tip of the stereotactic probe. The probe could also be used to record the electrical activity of the brain tissue through which it passed on the way to the target. This electrophysiologic recording became a valuable aid to accurate placement of the needle. With such refinements in technique, the stereotactic surgeons were able to limit the damage to a very small volume of brain tissue, of the order of several cubic millimeters. In experienced hands such as those of Dr. Narabayashi, extremely precise operations were possible, tailored precisely to the needs of the individual patient.

These techniques were used to operate on many thousands of patients at special centers throughout the world. Although these operations effectively reduced tremor and rigidity on one side of the body in most cases, they nevertheless stirred considerable controversy. No one could satisfactorily explain why the operations worked. Many thoughtful physicians were disturbed by the idea of treating a disease whose symptoms reflected some poorly understood brain dysfunction by injuring the brain and causing further change in function, which was also poorly understood. Brain surgery could not cure or even alter the future progress of Parkinson's disease, and it relieved only some symptoms, mainly tremor and rigidity. Moreover, the operation had to be done twice, once for each side, if the symptoms on both sides of the body were to be relieved; and complications were much more frequent when both sides were operated on.

The major risk of stereotactic brain surgery was the possibility that the needle, pushed blindly through the brain toward the desired target, might injure a blood vessel and cause bleeding or clotting. The result would in effect be a stroke. There was also some difficulty because the standard measurement did not apply to all individuals, and as a result the needle might be placed a few millimeters off the target. Weakness of the arm or leg occasionally resulted, and in some the operation failed to give appreciable or lasting relief of tremor.

With experienced neurosurgeons the results were generally good and the risks relatively small. The chance of dying as a result of the operation was less than 1%. There was a 2% to 3% chance of some permanent weakness of the hand or leg on one side. Tremor and rigidity were markedly alleviated in 70% to 80% of cases. The results were less favorable when the second side was operated on. Especially troublesome was the development of slurring of speech and difficulty swallowing after the second operation. This occurred in as many as 15% to 20% of patients who were operated on twice.

To minimize risks, the surgeons were cautious in choosing patients on whom to operate. Not surprisingly, the best results were obtained in young patients whose symptoms were mainly on one side and who were in good general health. Complications were more frequent in the elderly and especially in patients who had high blood pressure, diabetes, arteriosclerosis, heart disease, or other disorders affecting general health. It was also found that patients who had severe bradykinesia were not as likely to benefit from the operation as those who had only tremor and rigidity. Impairment of equilibrium during walking was not helped and sometimes was made worse. Speech dysfunction was not improved by surgery. Patients who were severely affected with Parkinson's disease were not likely to experience improvement.

As the neurosurgeons who specialized in this type of surgery gained experience, they narrowed their criteria for selecting patients for surgery. The criteria eventually became rather strict, so that even the most aggressive and enthusiastic surgeons found only approximately 10% of Parkinson patients suitable for surgery. In the remaining 90%, the risks of surgery were considered too great and the likelihood of real benefit too small. Thus, despite all the publicity it received, stereotactic surgery was rather disappointing for many patients and their doctors.

There is no denying that early stereotactic surgery did help many patients and that the results were occasionally dramatic. The operations were performed under local anesthesia with the patient awake throughout the procedure. Many patients described with wonderment and awe how they felt when the tremor suddenly stopped during the surgery. Margaret Bourke White, a famous photographer, gave an excellent subjective account. She wrote magazine articles and later a book about her experience of Parkinson's disease and her operation (*The Autobiography of Margaret Bourke White*. Boston: G.K. Hall).

The publicity the operations received as a result of such individual accounts was a frequent cause of disappointment to the many patients who were not considered suitable for surgery. They had been led to hope for a miraculous cure by uncritical reports that appeared frequently in the popular press and in television documentaries. They sometimes had difficulty understanding why they too could not be helped. Many patients who were operated on and enjoyed good relief of tremor and rigidity were also disappointed when similar symptoms appeared in the opposite limbs several years later. They had hoped that the operation would cure the disease or at least prevent its further progression. But, in fact, stereotactic surgery was nothing more than a symptomatic remedy for tremor and rigidity. It was not specific for Parkinson's disease but could alleviate these symptoms in many other conditions. Indeed, it is especially effective in relieving essential tremor.

In the past decade, the earlier pallidotomy procedure has received renewed attention as a result of the work of Drs. L. Laitinen in Sweden and Mahlon DeLong at Emory University in Atlanta. Dr. Laitinen felt that the operation relieved not only tremor and rigidity but also to some extent bradykinesia. Dr. DeLong's studies of the physiology of the basal ganglia in monkeys have given us new insight into the workings of this mysterious part of the brain and its dysfunction in Parkinson's disease. His work led him to the conclusion that pallidotomy was more effective than thalamotomy. He developed a new approach, based on careful recording of electrical activity in the pallidum, that defines the area of greatest abnormality within the pallidum; the object of surgery then is to destroy that small region. His data show that without the electrical recording, one can miss the area of abnormal activity and thus fail to do much good for the patient. This work has stimulated renewed interest in stereotactic brain surgery in the treatment of parkinsonism. As a result, pallidotomy is now being offered at a number of centers. Although the number of patients undergoing this new technique is not very large, the results do appear to be useful in well-selected cases.

Dr. Jean Siegfreid of Zurich, Switzerland; Dr. Alim Benabid of Grenoble, France; and others have studied the effects of direct electrical stimulation of the thalamus and other nuclei (globus pallidum and subthalamic nucleus) in the treatment of essential tremor and parkinsonism. They implant a fine wire electrode into the desired region of the brain. The wire is left in place and connected to a battery-driven stimulator. The idea is that high-frequency stimulation of the nucleus may "jam" the nerve circuits involved and thus mimic the effects of destructive lesions. The results are encouraging and stimulation procedures are now gaining prominence in the treatment of Parkinson's disease. (See the following section for more details.)

Many patients who may be expected to benefit from an operation choose not to undergo surgery. It is a personal choice that should be made rationally, with full understanding of the possible benefits and risks. An example is a long-time patient, Mrs. S., a pleasant 55-year-old woman who had a mild resting tremor in her left hand and foot. It did not interfere with her life or her work as a cashier. The tremor disappeared with levodopa treatment only to be replaced by constant involuntary writhing movements of the left hand and foot, which Mrs. S. found just as disagreeable as the tremor. Other medications gave only slight relief. After trying various doses and schedules, she finally decided to give up on levodopa. The involuntary movements stopped, but the tremor recurred exactly as before. Twenty years after her tremor first appeared, she still had no symptom other than tremor of her left hand and foot. It had become slightly more prominent over the years and at times affected her chin, but there was no tremor on the right side or other symptoms of Parkinson's disease. Mrs. S. retired at age 70 and subsequently lived a happy and very active life doing the many things she had dreamed of doing during the years she was working. She remained unwilling to have brain surgery even though chances were very good that her tremor could have been stopped.

Mrs. S. illustrates an important limitation of stereotactic surgery in the treatment of parkinsonism. One symptom that this surgery can most effectively relieve, regardless of its cause, is tremor, but patients who have only tremor and no other symptoms are rarely interested in having brain surgery. It is later in the course of Parkinson's disease, when slowness of movement, poor equilibrium, difficulty walking, and other, more disturbing symptoms appear, that most patients are willing to undergo surgery. Unfortunately, not all of these more serious symptoms are appreciably helped by stereotactic surgery—and some symptoms may even be made worse. Thus, when the patients really need help, surgery may not be effective. Although thalamic, pallidal, or subthalamic nucleus surgery would almost certainly have benefited Mrs. S., one cannot argue with her decision. It was hers to make, and she remained confident that she made the right choice.

It is therefore important to realize that surgery is not a treatment for parkinsonism generally to be used in all patients. It is most useful in dealing with certain symptoms that do not respond to or are made worse by drug treatment. For example, painful muscle spasms may develop in a leg or arm and worsen with continued drug treatment. These spasms prevent the patient from getting a good effect from drug treatment. Surgery can relieve these spasms and allow the patient to obtain better results from anti-Parkinson medications. But surgery usually will not benefit patients unable to stand or walk due to lack of equilibrium or marked freezing. In the following section, we will outline the various types of surgery and their uses.

SURGICAL PROCEDURES AND INDICATIONS

Surgery should be considered only after all reasonable medical options have been tried and have proved inadequate to control the symptoms and complications of Parkinson's disease. The complications of surgery can be devastating, including stroke, bleeding in the brain, seizures, confusion, speech abnormalities, worsening of the target symptoms, and even death. The total complication rate varies widely from study to study, but it is not unfair to say that it hovers around 15% in the best of hands. Many surgical complications do prove to be transitory but certainly not all, as is evident from the nature of those listed earlier.

Much of what we will say in the following paragraphs comes from studies of surgical outcomes directed by Dr. Anthony Lang, Professor of Neurology at the University of Toronto. It is to his careful research that we owe much of our recent knowledge about the indications and uses of the various surgical procedures.

Surgical procedures can be divided into two major categories: (a) ablative lesions and (b) deep brain stimulation. Ablative lesioning means that the surgeon puts an electrode into the target nucleus of the brain (see the list of current target nuclei that follows) and burns out a small part of the area, killing all the cells in that immediate vicinity. The surgeon then removes the electrode, leaving no devices or hardware in the patient's body. These lesions (destruction of cells) are permanent and, once completed, cannot be undone. Deep brain stimulation (DBS) means that the surgeon puts an electrode into a specific target nucleus but leaves the electrode in place. The electrode is attached to a stimulator underneath the patient's chest skin (similar to what is done with a heart pacemaker) that can be turned on or off at will. One can think of such stimulation as temporarily exhausting the cells in the local area of stimulation to the point where they are not functioning. The net result therefore is the same as that with ablative lesion. The area of stimulation can be adjusted by programming the stimulator after it is in place. Such adjustment allows the surgeon to change the size and severity of the lesion and even allows the location of the lesion to be changed slightly, if necessary. The stimulator can be turned on all the time, or used only for certain hours during the day when needed. It is therefore a much more flexible approach than simple ablative lesions. It is also a much more complex process, requiring permanent hardware in the brain and body.

Currently, there are three targets for both ablative lesions and DBS: (a) the thalamus, (b) the internal globus pallidus, and (c) the subthalamic nucleus. Each target has its particular indications and uses. Choosing the best location therefore becomes a very important neurologic and surgical decision. Since DBS or ablative lesions can in theory be performed in all three of these target nuclei, choosing the best procedure is also a very important decision that must be made for each patient individually. These decisions need to be made by a team consisting of a neurologist and neurosurgeon working together in a Parkinson's disease center.

The thalamus is a good target to relieve tremor. Ablative lesioning (thalamotomy) has about a 90% success rate and the effect tends to be long lasting. Rigidity or stiffness may be helped somewhat in 40% of patients but the major disabling problems associated with slowness (bradykinesia) or walking do not really respond at all. Therefore, thalamotomy or thalamic stimulation is reserved for those with disabling tremor only. Significant complications of thalamic lesions include weakness on the opposite side of the body, slurred speech, confusion, or even increased tremor on the same side of the body as the lesion.

Lesions of the internal globus pallidus (pallidotomy and pallidal stimulation) are most useful in diminishing abnormal involuntary movements (dyskinesias) on the opposite side of the body. Patients with disabling levodopa-induced dyskinesias are therefore good candidates for pallidal surgery. Fluctuations tend to improve with pallidal lesions. Patients with major disability during their off periods (when levodopa is not working) may benefit with improvement of slowness and to a lesser degree rigidity, walking, and tremor. The benefit to tremor is not nearly as good as that with thalamic lesions. Interestingly, however, Parkinson's symptoms often, but not always, improve considerably on both sides of the body even if only one side of the brain is lesioned. If a patient has undergone an ablative lesion (pallidotomy) on one side of the brain and does require additional surgery to relieve symptoms on the other side of the body, it is currently recommended that the second surgery be deep brain stimulation of the globus pallidus or subthalamic nucleus rather than a second pallidotomy. Ablative lesions on both sides of the brain are associated with more side effects than single-sided lesions.

For all practical purposes, lesioning of the subthalamic nucleus is achieved with DBS only. Except in extraordinary cases, ablative lesioning is considered too risky. The advantage of this target is that lesions here benefit many more of the disabling symptoms of Parkinson's disease: stiffness, dyskinesias, slowness, motor fluctuations, and tremor. Unfortunately, complications can also be significant and include muscular contractions, slurred speech, pins-and-needles sensation, eye deviations, mental changes (including confusion), infections and various types of hardware breakdowns. The current procedure is to contemplate doing subthalamic DBS on both sides of the brain, although the electrodes may be placed one at a time at two separate operations.

It must be remembered that surgery in its present state is neither a cure nor a final therapeutic endpoint. It should be considered a late therapeutic option for appropriate candidates. Some patients respond well to surgery; others, less well. Nevertheless, particularly with current deep brain stimulation procedures performed with proper testing and by experienced surgeons, surgical intervention is a valuable addition to the armamentarium in the fight against the progressive symptoms of Parkinson's disease.

BRAIN TRANSPLANTS

The surgical treatment of Parkinson's disease took a new twist in the 1980s with attempts to transplant dopamine-producing nerve cells into the corpus striatum. The idea was to replace the lost dopamine-producing nerve cells of the substantia nigra with new ones placed directly in the striatum where the substantia nigra nerve cells normally deliver their dopamine. One source of such cells is the adrenal gland. Although the cells of the adrenal gland chiefly produce adrenaline (epinephrine), they also produce some dopamine. A better source of dopamine-producing nerve cells is the region of the midbrain where the substantia nigra is located. Using a microscope, researchers were able to dissect out this region from fetal or newborn animals and transplant it into the striatum of an adult animal. The nerve cells in these transplants survived, grew, and proved capable of at least partially correcting experimentally induced parkinsonism in rats, marmosets, and monkeys.

Building on this experience with transplants in rats, a Swedish group attempted adrenal-to-brain transplants in four Parkinson's disease patients from 1981 to 1984. The results were disappointing, and they concluded that this approach held little promise. However, a neurosurgeon in Mexico, Dr. Ignaccio Madrazzo, reported dramatic benefits with adrenal transplants in human patients. The first two patients were young, 33 and 35 years of age, and their parkinsonism atypical so that it was not clear what disease they had. One patient did so well that he no longer needed levodopa! Dr. Madrazzo's reports stirred great interest, and within a year a number of American surgeons also attempted adrenal transplants in Parkinson patients. They thought that some differences in technique might have accounted for the better results reported by the Mexican surgeon. Within a short time, several hundred patients had this surgery. However, the procedure required two major operations performed one immediately after the other: the first to remove an adrenal gland and the second to implant a portion of the gland into the striatum. This was a considerable stress on older patients weakened by Parkinson's disease. Not surprisingly, there were a substantial number of serious complications and some deaths. The results proved disappointing. No one could reproduce the dramatic initial results claimed by Madrazzo. The reason became apparent when several patients were subsequently studied postmortem. It was found that the transplanted adrenal nerve cells had not survived. The pathologists found a mass of dead and dying adrenal cells surrounded by inflammatory cells at the transplant site.

Both the initial claims of success and the subsequent disappointment received wide coverage in the public media. The American Academy of Neurology and other organizations called for a halt to the transplant operations until the results could be fully evaluated. A careful follow-up evaluation of a large number of cases in 1989 by a group of neurologists led by Drs. Christopher Goetz of the Rush–Presbyterian–St. Luke's Medical Center in Chicago, Warren Olanow of the University of South Florida (now at Mount Sinai School of Medicine in New York); and William Koller of the University of Kansas (now at the University of Miami School of Medicine) found that benefits had been minimal and were not sustained. Adrenal transplants were abandoned.

FETAL-TISSUE TRANSPLANTS

Meanwhile, a Swedish group led by Dr. Olle Lindval at the University of Lund began a long-term study of the effects of human fetal-cell transplants in human patients in a careful and methodical manner. They operated on their first patient in 1987 and the second in 1988. They have since proceeded very slowly, carefully evaluating the results and improving their techniques at each step. They learned that early the best results occurred when the transplant was placed in the region of the striatum called the putamen, where the loss of dopamine is the greatest in Parkinson's disease. All patients were also treated with drugs to suppress the immune system.

By 1994, they had operated on only 16 patients, including two who had parkinsonism induced by N-methylphenyl tetrahydropyridine (MPTP), a contaminant in illicit "street" drugs. Dr. Lindval reported the results at the third international meeting of the Movement Disorders Society in Orlando, Florida, in December 1994. This was the most extensive assessment then available of the possibilities of this type of transplant surgery. Improvements first appeared about 5 to 6 months after the operation and continued for up to 2 to 5 years. Improvement in on–off fluctuations with increased "on" time and less severe "off" periods was observed in five of the first 10 patients. Gait impairments were improved in two patients. One patient showed no response to the surgery, and Dr. Lindval believes the diagnosis of Parkinson's disease was probably incorrect. A reduction in levodopa dosage was possible in some cases. However, new symptoms also appeared, reflecting progression of the disease. Most patients had the transplant surgery on only one side of the brain, so the improvements were seen on the opposite side of the body; Parkinson symptoms continued to progress on the same side of the body as the surgery was performed. Poor balance developed in one patient, and as we have noted, this symptom is not always responsive to levodopa treatment and may not be due to dopamine deficiency.

In an international collaboration, Swedish patients with fetal grafts were studied at the Hammersmith Hospital in London to check on the progress of the graft. The studies involved an imaging method known as positron emission tomography (PET) (more fully described on pages 150–151). The PET scans have shown that the transplanted cells survive and are able to take up levodopa and convert it to dopamine. Repeat PET scans showed that the transplants grew slowly and then remained about the same size 3 to 4 years after the transplantation. However, the scans also showed that the patients' own dopamine systems deteriorated during this period. The dopamine cells in the graft are apparently doing well, but the patients' own dopamine brain cells continue to deteriorate as expected. This indicates that whatever causes dopamine nerve cells to deteriorate does not affect the grafted cells.

A number of other surgical teams have attempted fetal brain transplants, including a group led by Dr. Curt Freed at the University of Colorado, collaborating with Dr. Stanley Fahn at Columbia University in a study sponsored by the National Institutes of Health to assess the benefits of the transplant procedure in 40 patients. The patients had the surgery at the University of Colorado and were studied in New York at Columbia University. One-half the study patients had a sham procedure. That is, an operation was done but no graft was implanted. Neither the evaluating doctors nor the patients knew which patients received the graft. Both were thus "blind" to the treatment given. This "double-blind" procedure assured a reasonably objective assessment of the graft procedure. The results were mixed and probably should be considered disappointing. Older patients did not respond. Patients under 60 years of age may have had a response. A major long-term complication seems to be "runaway" dyskinesias in which involuntary movements become increasingly uncontrollable with time.

Difficult ethical and troubling moral questions surround the use of living human tissue obtained from aborted fetuses. Guidelines have been formulated by various scientific and professional bodies for the procurement, handling, and use of human fetal tissue. They draw from the guidelines developed over many years for human organ transplants. However, the use of fetal tissue is not strictly comparable to collecting organs from brain-dead patients or cadavers. Since fetal tissue can only be acquired from aborted fetuses, many find the approach morally unacceptable. The ethical and moral objections to the use of fetal cells could be circumvented by using artificial or genetically engineered cells maintained in tissue cultures. Many "lines" of such cells exist and some have already been shown to alleviate parkinsonism in animals with MPTP-induced parkinsonism. Transplantation with a patient's own cells that have been genetically engineered to act like dopamine-producing cells offers another approach for future therapy. Such cells have not yet been transplanted into human patients. Another approach has been to consider transplanting animal cells to the brains of patients with Parkinson's disease. There is currently a great deal of concern about using such cells, particularly cells of pig brain. Pig brain cells may contain viruses capable of causing serious infections of the brain, suppression of the immune system, or even cancer. We believe, however, that advances in other areas, especially the genetic aspects of Parkinson's disease, will lead to entirely new and more effective treatments than those offered by transplantation strategies.

12

Dietary Considerations

Malnutrition can cause disturbances—even very serious disturbances—of the nervous system, including various paralyses, loss of feeling, incoordination, convulsions, and mental deterioration; but malnutrition has never caused parkinsonism. No known nutritional deficiency is responsible for or characteristic of parkinsonism.

Nor, aside from levodopa, is there any known food or special nutrient, vitamin, or mineral that has a therapeutic effect. Consequently, there is no dietary treatment. Contrary to what one may read in magazine articles or popular books on nutrition, no diet or food is known to have a beneficial effect on the symptoms of Parkinson's disease or other forms of parkinsonism.

The best dietary advice for patients with parkinsonism is to eat as normally as possible. The patient should attend to his or her general health and should eat a well-balanced diet with fruits, vegetables, adequate protein, roughage, cereal, and so on.

Since a tendency to constipation is common in Parkinson patients, special attention to roughage and natural laxatives is warranted. Many patients find it beneficial to eat prunes or figs regularly. Roughage and high-fiber foods such as carrots, cauliflower, broccoli, bran cereals, and so on, are helpful in increasing the bulk of the stool. Patients who tend to have small, hard, "rocklike" stools should also make an effort to drink more water. A regimen of four to eight glasses a day—to be taken even if one does not feel thirsty—should be followed. Observing these simple, well-known, effective principles can appreciably reduce the need for laxatives. Unfortunately, many patients seem to prefer to resort to laxatives rather than to follow these more natural practices. Thus the best results are found in patients who have a concerned spouse able to encourage, constantly remind, and even scold as needed.

We mentioned earlier that a meal rich in protein, such as a hearty steak dinner, tends to reduce the absorption of levodopa. If levodopa is taken after such a meal, it is poorly absorbed and the therapeutic effect may be diminished. Some dietitians recommend that patients avoid excessive protein intake and limit themselves to the recommended dietary allowance of 56 g per day for men or 46 g for women. This is a very small amount of protein—less than that found in an ordinary one-quarter-pound hamburger.

The tendency of protein to interfere with levodopa therapy suggests that low-protein diets might be useful. In fact, such diets have repeatedly been studied as possible adjuncts to levodopa therapy. The results are clear: Levodopa is better absorbed on a low-protein diet—so much so that symptoms of overdosage may occur if the dose is not reduced. A smaller dose yields the same blood level and the same results when the patient is on a low-protein diet as a larger dose when the patient is on a normal diet. Unfortunately, the results are otherwise similar. There seems to be no definite advantage in the low-protein diet. Moreover, it is difficult to make very-low-protein diets palatable. Patients soon tire of them and revert to their customary eating habits. Dr. Jonathan Pincus of Georgetown University Medical School in Washington, DC, has advocated a diet confining protein to the evening meal for patients with fluctuations in their response to levodopa treatment. The diet does reduce "off" episodes during the day. Although some patients have found it useful, in our experience the benefits are minimal, and the patients tire of the diet after a month or two. Several low-protein prepared food products in packets and cans have been marketed recently to Parkinson patients, with the claim of providing a nutritionally balanced and tasty diet that can aid patients with motor fluctuations gain a better control of symptoms. In our experience, the best course is to adjust the dosage to the patient's customary diet, but then the diet should be consistent. Meals should be at regular times. Gastronomic excesses should be avoided.

There is no reason to forbid the use of alcoholic beverages in normal amounts. Those who are accustomed to having a glass of wine at dinner need not abandon this custom. Patients who enjoy a glass of beer or a cocktail in the evening or at a social occasion need not be deprived of this pleasure. Moderation and common sense are the watchwords here. Excesses should be carefully avoided.

Alcoholism seems to be very rare among Parkinson patients. There seems to be something about Parkinson's disease that protects against this all too common scourge. The reason is not known.

In this day of popular dietary foods, "megavitamins," "natural" foods, and health food stores, a few words about these foods in respect to parkinsonism seem in order. Generally, there is no reason the Parkinson patient may not partake of these currently popular dietary fads if he or she so desires. However, there should be no hope that such foods or megavitamins can influence the disease. Some may be "good" in the sense that they are nutritious and thus "good" for anybody, but they are not beneficial specifically for people with Parkinson's disease.

Vitamins are substances required by the body in minute, or trace, amounts. Deficiency of the known vitamins can cause serious disturbances. Specific deficiency diseases are known for each vitamin: Scurvy results from vitamin C deficiency, beriberi from vitamin B_1 deficiency, rickets from vitamin D deficiency, and so on. If the Parkinson patient has no deficiency and eats a normal diet, taking supplemental vitamins is useless. Contrary to popular belief, vitamins do not supply "pep" or energy or strength. They are taken as a sort of insurance against some possible deficiency due to poor eating habits. It is probably a good idea for older people generally to take a multiple vitamin tablet daily, especially since the elderly often eat poorly. There is nothing specific about Parkinson patients that makes them susceptible to vitamin deficiencies. However, there is an interesting story about vitamin B_6 (pyridoxine) and parkinsonism that we might do well to review briefly.

THE PYRIDOXINE STORY

Vitamin B_6 (pyridoxine) was recommended for the treatment of parkinsonism shortly after it was first discovered about 1938. It proved ineffective, and in 1950 the American Medical Association's Council on Pharmacy consulted leading experts on the subject and concluded that pyridoxine had no place in the treatment of parkinsonism. However, pyridoxine is known to be essential for the optimal function of the enzyme that controls the chemical conversion of L-dopa (and levodopa) to dopamine in the body. For this reason, when the deficiency of brain dopamine in Parkinson's disease was first discovered, there was renewed interest in pyridoxine. It was tried again in the treatment of parkinsonism in large doses: 1 g per day or so, approximately 1,000 times more than the daily dose recommended for nutritional purposes. Again, no effect was noted. Nevertheless, the notion that pyridoxine was good for those with Parkinson's disease persists among some nutritionists; accordingly, they recommend that foods known to be rich in vitamin B_6 be included in the diet. These include wheat germ, bran, brewer's yeast, tomatoes, liver, and soybeans. Brewer's yeast is very rich in vitamin B_6 and has been recommended for Parkinson patients. These foods are perfectly fine for anyone to eat, and Parkinson patients may certainly eat heartily of them. However, no one has ever presented any evidence that patients eating these foods fare any better than patients who do not. Since pyridoxine, even in doses far larger than the amount available in foods, has been found ineffective in treating parkinsonism, it seems unlikely that foods rich in vitamin B_6 could be helpful.

In the early days of levodopa, research physicians added pyridoxine in the expectation that they would thereby enhance its conversion to dopamine. There seemed to be no advantage in doing so. In fact, to everyone's surprise, it proved deleterious. It was found that adding pyridoxine canceled out all the effects of levodopa. Patients doing well on levodopa who took "therapeutic" vitamins containing large amounts of pyridoxine suffered a gradual recurrence of their Parkinson symptoms within a week or two as if the levodopa were no longer working. When they stopped taking the vitamin pills, the levodopa gradually became effective again.

The reason pyridoxine has this effect on levodopa treatment is that the enzyme that converts levodopa to dopamine does its job so much faster in the presence of abnormally high amounts of vitamin B_6. It converts it all to dopamine before it can get a chance to reach the brain. Dopamine, alas, cannot enter the brain to reach the dopamine nerve cells of the substantia nigra. The drugs carbidopa and benserazide (see discussion in Chapter 7) have the opposite effect of pyridoxine: They inhibit the enzyme that converts levodopa to dopamine. Fortunately, they do not enter the brain and thus affect the formation of dopamine inside the brain. They prevent pyridoxine from reversing the effect of levodopa in parkinsonism. Thus patients being treated with combined levodopa–carbidopa (Sinemet) or levodopa–benserazide (Madopar) can eat anything they please and take all the vitamins they wish without risking "pyridoxine reversal." However, a word of caution is in order. The protection against pyridoxine reversal may not always be complete. Thus it would still be wise to avoid "therapeutic doses" or "mega-doses" of vitamins, unless they are really necessary and prescribed by a physician; the dose of vitamin B_6 should be less than 50 mg a day. Fortunately, very few conditions require treatment with large doses of vitamin B_6.

VITAMIN C

Vitamin C (ascorbic acid) has enjoyed a popular reputation as a preventive and treatment for the common cold ever since Linus Pauling claimed it was effective in preventing colds. Megadoses have been used: 0.5- or 1.0-g tablets one to several times daily. Whether or not vitamin C is effective in preventing colds need not concern us here. There seems to be no reason Parkinson patients may not take vitamin C in any reasonable dose. It might be used, for example, to acidify the urine in cases of bladder infection.

VITAMIN E

Vitamin E (α-tocopherol) has been widely promoted as being helpful in an immense variety of conditions. The large number of areas in which it has been claimed to be effective suggests that it is not effective in any. It was once widely used to relieve painful leg cramps, especially those occurring in sleep (nocturnal cramps). We have given it to Parkinson patients complaining of leg cramps, but it did not seem helpful in any. The patients sometimes thought it helped but ceased using it after a while. Some complained it made them drowsy and tired.

For theoretical reasons, it was suggested many years ago that vitamin E may retard aging and the progression of Parkinson's disease and Alzheimer's disease. It was speculated that oxygen ions, or "radicals," played a role in these diseases. Conclusive evidence that such is the case has been difficult to obtain. A national collaborative study called the DATATOP (*D*eprenyl *a*nd *T*ocopherol *A*ntioxidant *T*herapy *o*f *P*arkinsonism) study has objectively tested the possibility that vitamin E might retard the normal progression of Parkinson's disease (also see discussion in Chapter 5). High doses—2,000 international units (IU) per day—were used in the study. The results did not show any effect on the signs and symptoms of Parkinson's disease. There is no evidence that vitamin E has any value in ameliorating the symptoms of Parkinson's disease or slowing the disease progression.

Vitamin E deficiency has been found to be the cause of deterioration of peripheral nerves seen in patients with chronic intestinal malabsorption or an inherited abnormality of vitamin E metabolism. The symptoms include weakness or diminished sensation in the legs and unsteadiness in walking, but nothing resembling parkinsonism. In these patients, the blood level of vitamin E is very low.

As far as we know, vitamin E in reasonable doses is harmless, and there seems little reason to object to anyone using it who believes there is some benefit in it. The recommended dose is one 400-IU tablet daily.

VITAMIN B₁₂

Injections of vitamin B_{12} (cyanocobalamin) were formerly sometimes administered by physicians as a sort of "tonic." Many patients claimed that it made them feel stronger. Physicians may give it in the hope of relieving the sense of weakness or fatigue that is so common a complaint in Parkinson patients. However, there is no known reason or clear evidence that vitamin B_{12} injections are indeed helpful in dealing with these symptoms.

Deficiency in vitamin B_{12} results in a particular kind of anemia, termed *pernicious anemia*. Patients with this disorder cannot absorb vitamin B_{12} from the diet. If vitamin B_{12} deficiency is suspected, tests can be done to determine if in fact there is a deficiency. The amount in the blood can be measured. If a deficiency is found, its cause should be determined by appropriate tests, and treatment with vitamin B_{12} instituted. Otherwise, there is no recognized justification for vitamin B_{12} treatment in Parkinson patients.

MINERALS

Because of the tendency for bones to lose their calcium content gradually over the years, many physicians and nutritionists recommend supplemental mineral intake for the middle-aged and elderly, with particular attention to calcium.

Some iron solutions are often recommended, especially to menstruating women, to counter the loss of iron in menstrual blood. Iron deficiency leads to anemia, but in the absence of iron deficiency supplemental iron is useless. Iron deficiency anemia should be treated with large doses of iron, much larger than the amount in the usual vitamin tablet "fortified" with iron. In any event, iron has no therapeutic effect in parkinsonism and does not relieve the sense of fatigue or weakness, unless there is indeed an iron deficiency anemia. The physician can easily determine with a blood count whether the patient is anemic, and the amount of iron in the body can be determined by sending a tube of blood to the laboratory to measure its iron content. If iron deficiency is present, the doctor can treat it appropriately. If not, there is no need to take iron or iron-fortified vitamins. Iron, incidentally, tends to increase constipation.

Sodium chloride, the mineral sprinkled on food as common table salt, may be helpful in combating the low blood pressure some patients have on levodopa therapy. The doctor should prescribe the amount of salt. Usually, 1 or 2 g per day does the trick. This is much more of course than can be obtained by salting food heavily. Salt tablets in 0.5- and 1-g sizes are usually readily available in drug and grocery stores, especially during the summer. There are, however, potential medical complications of excessive salt intake. It may exacerbate high blood pressure, chronic congestive heart failure, and so on. Thus older people should let their doctor decide if they need to increase their salt intake.

AMINO ACID SUPPLEMENTS

The amino acid L-tryptophan was studied some years ago as a treatment for depression. Some evidence accumulated that in large doses (10 to 15 g per day) it can indeed relieve the common depression, or "involutional melancholia," of middle age. The dose required is considerably larger than the amount one could get by dietary manipulation. Purified L-tryptophan has been sold in health food stores as a "natural" sedative and tranquilizer, but used in these small doses, it has no definite effect.

L-Tryptophan is a naturally occurring amino acid and is a precursor of the chemical messenger serotonin in much the same way that levodopa is the precursor of dopamine. Both dopamine and serotonin are present in the corpus striatum in substantial amounts. The relationships between these two important chemical messengers in the brain is not yet fully understood, but there is some evidence of antagonism. Large doses of L-tryptophan have been reported to exacerbate parkinsonism, especially when combined with pyridoxine. L-Tryptophan has also been reported to diminish the severity of chorea, a condition that is in many ways the opposite of parkinsonism. Some clinicians advocated giving L-tryptophan to patients receiving levodopa to counter the side effects of the latter. However, we have found that, even when given in very large doses to Parkinson patients on levodopa therapy, it produced no effect on the parkinsonian state itself or on the side effects of levodopa.

It had been reported in various lay publications that L-tryptophan was beneficial for tremor. Some patients therefore obtained the amino acid at their local health food store and have taken it on their own. It is quite possible that the L-tryptophan is helpful in certain kinds of tremor, such as the severe tremulousness known as *action myoclonus,* but it is not helpful in parkinsonism.

In late 1989, the Centers for Disease Control of the U.S. Public Health Service officially recognized an epidemic of a strange malady in those taking L-tryptophan; it was called the *eosinophilia–myalgia syndrome.* Muscle aches and pains, weakness, and fatigue were the main symptoms. Cough, difficulty in breathing, skin rash, and swelling of the ankles also occurred in some cases. A marked increase in the number of "eosinophil cells" in the blood was found. These are a type of white blood cell that typically increases in allergic reactions. This toxic reaction was thought to result from an impurity.

CHOLINE AND LECITHIN

Dopamine is not the only chemical messenger affected by the ingestion of its precursor. For example, the amount of acetylcholine formed in the brain can be increased by feeding its precursor choline. Supplementing the diet with large amounts of choline chloride (10 to 15 g daily) can suppress the involuntary movements in certain types of chorea. Choline can at least partially and transiently correct impairment of recent memory in some patients afflicted with senile mental deterioration or with Alzheimer's disease.

For several years, many people obtained choline in the form of choline tartrate at health food stores or over the counter at drugstores and pharmacies in the hope of improving their mental function. There is no evidence that choline can actually do this in the doses used. There is a good reason to be cautious about the use of choline in Parkinson patients. In view of the reciprocal, seesaw relationship between dopamine and acetylcholine (see discussion in Chapter 5), one might expect that increasing the formation of acetylcholine in the brain would exacerbate the parkinsonian state. And, in fact, it does just that! Therefore, we do not advise patients to take choline. (See also the section on cholinergic drugs in Chapter 6.)

13

Common Sense About Exercise

Physical activity in amounts commensurate with one's ability and strength can make an important contribution to health and well-being. Activity is necessary to maintain the body's musculature. Unused muscles quickly atrophy.

Similarly, joints need to move through their normal range of motion every day. A joint that is not used soon becomes stiff and eventually suffers a permanent loss of function. The surrounding tissues become firm and fibrotic. The joint can ultimately become frozen in a fixed posture. The patient is then said to have a *contracture* of that joint. Thus constant activity is essential to keep our musculoskeletal system with its muscles, bones, and joints functioning properly. Exercise also improves the heart and the circulation. Increased breathing during physical activity improves aeration of the lungs. The urinary tract—including the kidneys, ureters, and bladder—functions better in the upright position and is thus benefited when the individual rises and moves about. It is a common observation that physically active people have less trouble with constipation than those who lead sedentary lives. Finally, physical activity has a good effect on the mind. It is relaxing, calming, and often provides a welcome change of ideas. A sense of satisfaction and well-being is a common experience following exercise.

These obvious truisms merit repetition here because, unfortunately, Parkinson patients tend gradually to withdraw from their usual activities. For various reasons, they seem to do less and less as time goes on and eventually retire to a sedentary existence if a conscious effort is not made to continue normal activities. They seem to suffer an inertia that is probably an expression of the bradykinesia of Parkinson's disease (described in greater detail in Chapter 3). To combat this tendency, it is a good idea to follow a regular routine to assure a reasonable amount of physical activity every day. Whatever the activity, it should be done daily, regularly, and in moderation. Sudden bursts of frenetic activity separated by long periods of indolence are to be deplored. A regular and constant level of activity is best. If this can be done without even thinking about it, if the patient's lifestyle includes a regular and moderate amount of physical activity, that is all to the good. The specific nature of the activity is unimportant. We are not discussing physical activity as a treatment but as a means of maintaining a degree of physical fitness. No amount of physical activity or specific type of exercise can alter the basic disease process in the nervous system. However, a patient who remains physically fit is better able to cope with the various symptoms of Parkinson's disease as the years go by. It is a matter of common experience that patients who keep physically fit fare better in the long run than those who do not.

Some patients are fortunate in having an occupation that involves some measure of physical activity. We know a horticulturist with Parkinson's disease who retired at the usual age of 65 years. He was able to remain active in his work after retirement, working as a consultant and maintaining his own large garden and raising new rhododendron hybrids. The physical activity involved in his work provided him with an excellent quality of exercise. This man was also very fortunate in being able to continue after retirement the work he had known and loved most of his life. Some patients have a hobby or avocation that similarly entails some appreciable amount of good physical activity: fishing, hiking, rock collecting, and so on. They should by all means continue these activities. How much and how often they can do so is unfortunately often limited by weather, opportunity, and the seasonal nature of some of these activities. One of our patients learned to be an amateur glider pilot shortly before the first symptoms of Parkinson's disease developed. He was able to continue this hobby for a number of years. Ultimately, he had to give up gliding because of disease progression, but in the meantime he had derived pleasure and satisfaction from it, as well as some excellent physical activity. Many patients obtain perfectly good exercise through the pursuit of less dramatic but equally satisfying activities such as tending their gardens, doing light carpentry and masonry, or performing other yard work around the house.

Obviously, those patients who are able to cultivate an interest in something that keeps both mind and body active are very fortunate. We wish it were possible for more patients to develop such interests. Since there are so many opportunities for leisure activities today, it is a tragedy that more patients seem unable to participate. Unfortunately, most patients have to carry out some program of exercise as a routine chore. It would be much better if it were fun to do, but exercise is sufficiently important that patients should faithfully do some every day as a duty to themselves, even if it seems dull. It is a good idea for many patients to have someone else monitor the performance of their daily exercise routine, whatever it may be. The patient's wife or husband, relative, or friend should see to it that it is done. The patient may need to be reminded. The monitor should be prepared to urge, coax, and even insist that the exercise be done. Spouses naturally resent the role of drill sergeant, but it is a fact that patients whose devoted spouses see to it that some daily physical activity is done and done properly fare much better than those who are allowed to lapse into sedentary and inactive lives, slumped all day before a television set.

Exercise machines, stationary bicycles, rowing machines, and similar devices are very popular, and many patients use them happily and with benefit. However, there is nothing specific about this type of indoor exercise. It is useful when one cannot get more natural exercise. All that is really necessary is to put every muscle and joint through its normal range of motion a few times every day. The exercise need not be intensive or of long duration. It should not be pushed to the point of exhaustion or discomfort.

Walking is an excellent and moderate exercise. The speed, duration, and terrain can be varied to suit the patient's ability and strength. It is not tiring. Indeed, many patients find walking refreshing and relaxing. It is a convenient form of exercise that can be done equally well in the city, suburbs, or country. One can make a point of walking every day in the course of doing certain errands, such as walking to the corner store to get the newspaper every day. The return walk can be by a circuitous route, perhaps a different one now and then to give some variety. Walking a mile a day is a reasonable and quite common goal. Some patients find this too mild an exercise. Others can walk considerable distances in the pursuit of some hobby. One patient for many years walked throughout the city of New York to satisfy his interest in historical buildings. Another walked extensively through the fields and woodlands of New Jersey, collecting and studying wild flowers and becoming something of an expert on the wild flowers of the area. Another patient, an admitted "physical fitness nut," jogs every morning. He had been jogging for years before Parkinson's disease developed and continued this habit. More than 15 years later, he still jogs a mile every morning. This vigorous exercise has no doubt greatly benefited him, but we would not routinely recommend jogging to all patients and would not advise it for older patients who are not accustomed to it.

Swimming is also an excellent exercise. Patients who were good swimmers in earlier years may find this a satisfying activity. Of course, they need regular access to a suitable facility, preferably one available throughout the year. Swimming must be done under adequate supervision. Patients subject to recurrent episodes of bradykinesia may suddenly find themselves in serious trouble in the water should they suddenly freeze and be unable to function. Patients with significant disturbances of equilibrium and walking should also avoid water activities. They are likely to have difficulties wading in shallow water and often have trouble controlling their bodies when swimming in deep water. They may need to be rescued by a lifeguard. It is a cardinal rule of water safety that no one should swim alone. The best of swimmers heed this rule, for they realize that they are not immune to having a cramp or some other accident in the water. Certainly, Parkinson patients cannot ignore this rule.

Patients who have athletic skills in various sports such as tennis, golf, or squash should continue these activities. Of course, they can rarely be done on a daily basis and thus cannot be the only activity used for exercise. However, the pursuit of a learned skill is an excellent way to get healthful exercise.

Learned or acquired skills are apt to be less affected by parkinsonism than automatic instinctive activities such as walking. Thus patients who are able to continue a sport of this type requiring considerable motor skill can enjoy a quality of exercise that would otherwise be difficult if not impossible for them to obtain in other activities. Experienced mountain climbers, water skiers, acrobats, and so on should by all means continue their activities within reason and safely within their capabilities and the limitations imposed by parkinsonism.

CALISTHENICS

Some people have cultivated the habit of doing calisthenic exercises as a daily ritual, usually on arising in the morning or on retiring in the evening. Those with Parkinson's disease should certainly continue this excellent habit. Of course, age and general health are important factors that determine which exercises can be done. Obviously, push-ups, skipping rope, or jogging are too strenuous for elderly persons or those with heart disease or arthritis. Those with a diminished exercise tolerance may do simpler exercises, however, such as bicycling motions with the legs, circling movements with the arms, bending movements, and perhaps even squatting and sitting-up exercises. These various movements may be described as active range-of-motion exercises. They ensure that every large joint and its related muscles are put through their full range of motion. Repeated five to ten times or more in a systematic way, these exercises can be very helpful in maintaining physical fitness.

We hesitate to recommend any specific set of exercises for so diverse a group of people as the population of Parkinson patients who may come across these pages. However, for the average patient 50 to 70 years of age whose symptoms are reasonably well controlled by proper medical treatment, the following simple calisthenics may be suggested. Many patients find these too mild and wish to do more. Others may find one or two of these exercises too strenuous or difficult. The patient should consult a physician before embarking on these exercises to be sure there are no medical reasons for not doing them. In any case, these are offered simply to illustrate the type of exercises that many patients find helpful. Usually they are done in the morning on first arising, but they can of course be done at any time. No exercise should be continued that causes pain or discomfort or seems too difficult.

1. While lying flat on your back in bed, slowly lift one leg, knee bent, as high as you can. Then straighten the leg until the toes point to the ceiling. Hold this position for 30 to 60 seconds; then slowly lower the leg to the surface of the bed. Repeat five to ten times, first with one leg, then with the other.

2. Lying flat on your back, bend your head slowly to the right to bring the ear close to the shoulder; then slowly bend to the left in the same manner. Repeat ten times in each direction.
3. Still lying flat on your back, clasp your hands behind your head and try to sit up. Repeat five times. (This may be too difficult for some patients.)
4. Turn over to lie on your stomach. Place your hands behind your back; then lift the head, look up to the ceiling, and try to lift the chest off the surface of the bed. Now turn your head to the right and to the left, five times in each direction.
5. Sit up on the side of the bed, feet on the floor, and place hands on hips. Lean forward as far as possible, then lean backward but do not fall back onto the bed. Sit up straight, then lean first to the left, then to the right until the elbows touch the surface of the bed. Repeat five to ten times.
6. Stand up straight with hands on hips, head held high, shoulders back, and chest thrown forward. March in place 20 steps. Be sure to raise the knees up high and count out loud.
7. Stand erect, raise arms out to side, bringing hands to the level of the shoulders. Then raise arms and bring hands together over your head. Slowly lower arms to the horizontal, pulling the shoulders as far back as possible. Finally, lower arms to the side. Repeat five times.
8. Stand erect. Then bend forward from the hips in a relaxed manner. Allow the arms to fall downward, your hands hanging limply, fingers pointing to the floor. Do not force yourself to touch your toes with your fingers. This usually happens easily after you have done this exercise a number of times. Stand up straight. Repeat ten times.

Gentle, sensible exercises for older persons are illustrated in various videotapes. One we especially like is the program prepared by Angela Lansbury, the well-known actress and star of the television serial "Murder She Wrote." Many of her exercises should be useful to Parkinson patients.

THERAPEUTIC EXERCISES

We have been discussing activities and exercises of a general nature, useful to anyone—not only patients with Parkinson's disease—interested in maintaining physical fitness. There are, however, certain types of exercises that may be done with the aim of helping patients deal with specific Parkinson symptoms, such as stooped posture, the tendency to shuffle on walking, trouble getting up out of deep chairs, or the various other difficulties these patients have when carrying out ordinary tasks of daily life. Ideally, therapeutic exercises should be prescribed by a physiatrist—a physician trained in the medical specialty of physical medicine and rehabilitation—and should be performed by the patient under the supervision of a physical therapy nurse or technician, usually called a physical therapist. Most community hospitals have a department of physical medicine and rehabilitation where physical therapy can be obtained on a doctor's referral. Physical therapists may also provide treatment in freestanding facilities on a doctor's prescription. For those who are homebound, periodic visits by a physical therapist to instruct the patient in the exercises can be very helpful. The patient, however, must do the exercises at home alone every day, preferably under the watchful eye of his or her spouse, relative, or friend. Often the patient needs some assistance to perform certain exercises. At the next visit, the therapist can check the progress achieved, see that the patient is still doing the exercises properly, and modify the exercises or suggest new ones as needed. The therapist can reinforce the patient's performance by repeating the instruction and supervising the actual performance of the exercises.

The best exercises are *active* exercises done by the patient. The role of the therapist visiting the patient at home is mainly to see that the patient knows how to do the exercises and that an appropriate program of activities is being done. If necessary, the therapist can also administer passive range-of-motion and stretch exercises that the patient cannot do alone. However, such exercises must be done daily. It is not practicable to have a therapist visit the home daily, so the spouse or someone else must learn to do this type of physical treatment if it is needed. The therapist can teach the technique.

The following exercises are frequently recommended for specific problems. These are only a few examples. The therapist can teach additional ones or modify these to meet the special needs and circumstances of each patient. They should be done regularly, every day. They may help only for a short time after each performance, but a cumulative beneficial effect can usually be discerned after weeks of diligently practicing them every day.

Exercises for Stooped Posture

Back up against a wall, making sure that heels, shoulders, and the back of the head all touch the wall. Stand in this position for 1 minute, then walk—or better yet, march—across the room, stepping high, and return to the wall. Turn about and back up against the wall again. Note how much you have slumped forward during your march across the room and back. Repeat the entire exercise five times in the morning and again five times in the evening (Fig. 11).

Stand facing the wall, raise your hands as high as possible, and lean forward, placing the palms of your hands on the wall. Slowly push your hands up the wall as far as you can reach, arching your neck and spine backward a little and stretching upward. Repeat five times twice a day.

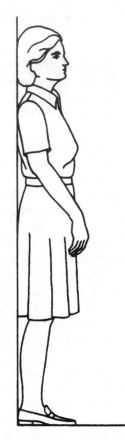

FIG. 11. Exercise for stooped posture.

Exercises for Shuffling and Festination

Practice walking or marching with high steps. Count a military-type marching cadence and keep time: "hup, two, three, four, left, right, left, right," and so on. Listen to the sounds of your feet striking the floor to get the rhythm.

If there is still difficulty raising the feet, place a series of books, magazines, wooden sticks, or other objects of similar size in a line across the room about one step apart. Step over these objects while marching across the room (Fig. 12).

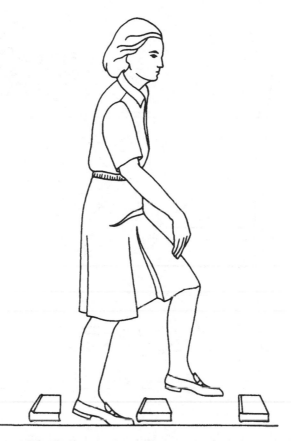

FIG. 12. Exercise for shuffling and festination.

Exercise for Sitting and Rising from Chairs

If you have particular trouble getting up out of chairs, practice sitting down and rising. Use a simple straight-backed chair. Study carefully the mechanics of sitting down and getting up out of a chair. To get up, slide forward on the seat, lean forward from the hips so that the trunk is inclined forward approximately 45 degrees, position your feet with one foot under the edge of the seat and the other a half step forward, and then place your hands on the sides of the seat near the front legs of the chair. Now push and step forward in one continuous, smooth motion (Fig. 13). If necessary, count to yourself: "one,

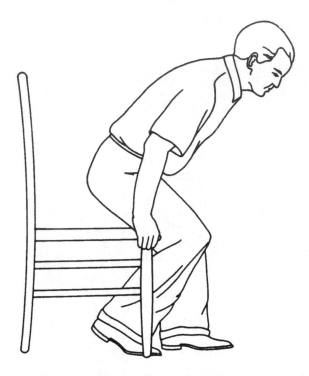

FIG. 13. Exercise for sitting and rising from chairs.

two, three, GO!" If you fail on the first attempt, rest a moment and try again. Try to get up suddenly before the Parkinson bradykinesia has a chance to block the movement.

To sit down, approach the chair briskly, turn about, then bend the trunk forward 45 degrees and sink down S L O W L Y onto the seat. Be careful to turn a sufficient amount to ensure that you end up properly centered on the seat. Try not to fall or slump into the chair. For practice, sit and rise five to ten times. Pay careful attention to each step in the sequence. A common failing is to sit down before turning about fully, with the result that the patient sits on one-half of the chair or misses the chair entirely and ends up on the floor. Proper footwork is the key. It helps if one foot is slightly behind the other and directly under the seat.

REHABILITATION SERVICES

Most patients need only practice a simple regimen of exercises on their own or with the help of their families to maintain a normal amount of physical activity. Some patients in addition may benefit from the occasional assistance of a physiatrist and a program of physical therapy with exercises along the lines of those just discussed. A small number of more severely affected patients who have problems carrying out the ordinary activities of daily life may need more intensive physical therapy to prevent invalidism. Special rehabilitation units for a thorough evaluation and a more intensive course of physical therapy are available in many communities at hospitals or free-standing outpatient clinics.

A patient who has deteriorated more rapidly than expected deserves a complete medical evaluation to make sure that some other disease process is not complicating the scene. The first indication that something else is going on—an ulcer, a kidney infection, a cancer, or some other serious illness—may be a patient's unexpectedly rapid decline over a period of months after doing quite well in controlling the symptoms of Parkinson's disease. If something is found, it may be possible to correct it and restore the patient to his or her former health.

Physical and occupational therapy can be given daily or several times per week, and every aspect of the patient's performance of daily living activities can be reviewed. Special training can then be given to teach the patient ways of overcoming the disabilities imposed by parkinsonism, and to eat, dress, bathe, comb, brush, and do the numerous ordinary tasks of daily life. In addition, intensive physical therapy can improve the patient's gait, posture, equilibrium, and performance of various motor acts.

After a course of therapy has been completed, every effort should be made to continue some physical therapy to maintain the benefits gained for as long as possible. The program of exercises must be carried out daily. A visit every week or two to the physical medicine department at the hospital or outpatient clinic serves to check progress and review the home exercise program. If necessary, arrangements can often be made to have a physical therapist visit the patient at home. The therapist may be able to make useful recommendations regarding the patient's life at home, the installation of hand rails and grab bars, and the use of various self-help devices. It may also be advisable to obtain some help at home. A part-time attendant or "home health aide" may be necessary to help the patient and family cope with the invalidism of advanced Parkinson's disease. The goal is to try to keep the patient at home and as independent as possible for as long as possible. The periodic visits of the visiting nurse service, if there is one in the area, may be very helpful. The visiting nurse can give valuable advice, help make arrangements for physical therapy, arrange transportation to the doctor's office or clinic, and provide home health aides and other medical social services.

Unfortunately, it is often difficult to convince the "third-party" organizations such as the Medicare carriers, Medicaid, and other health insurers to pay for physical therapy and other services at home for patients with chronic diseases. They do not seem to mind paying for such care to a patient recovering from a fracture or a stroke who needs therapy for only a limited time, but they are very reluctant to commit their funds and personnel to a course of therapy that may need to be continued indefinitely. They do not seem to understand that providing limited services at home, such as a weekly visit by a physical therapist and a visiting nurse, is in the long run a great deal better for the patient and a lot less expensive than the alternative of chronic care in a nursing home.

SUMMARY

Exercise has a definite place in the management of Parkinson's disease at every stage in its evolution. The choice of type of activity is a highly individual matter to be decided in consultation with the treating physician. In earlier stages of the disease, informal exercise and physical activity intended to maintain physical fitness are important. The problems that arise with more severe disease can be mitigated by specific exercises. Later, more intensive physical therapy may be required. Finally, even in the most advanced stages of the disease, some benefit is provided by physical therapy. Indeed, it is in the later and more severe stages of the disease that physical therapy can make its greatest contribution by preventing the complications of immobility. One final word of advice may be offered to all Parkinson patients on this general subject: Never give up any activity, never give up an inch of your independence until you absolutely must, for it is much more difficult to regain a lost activity than to hold onto it a little longer with the aid of some judicious exercise or physical therapy.

14

A Historical Perspective

Our present understanding of parkinsonism did not spring into being overnight but grew gradually over a long period of time, very slowly at first and then more and more rapidly. Most of our present knowledge was gained in the last 20 years. It has grown and changed appreciably even during the last few years. Doubtless it is changing, even as we write this passage, and will surely continue to change during the years ahead. It is thus impossible to give a final version of the truth about parkinsonism. It is not even possible to give the illusion that we can do so at this time because our knowledge and our concepts of the brain are evolving very rapidly. For this reason, as well as for putting some concepts in perspective, it is helpful to review briefly the history of our knowledge of parkinsonism.

The modern history of parkinsonism may be said to have begun in 1817, when James Parkinson published a small monograph, *An Essay on the Shaking Palsy.* In its pages, we find the first clear description of the condition we now call Parkinson's disease. The description is admittedly incomplete. Parkinson, a physician and surgeon practicing in London, had seen six cases over a period of some time. He was able to examine only one of these. It must be remembered here that the physical examination carried out by the modern medical practitioner had not yet been developed. None of the clinical techniques needed for evaluating the nervous system were then known. Neither the stethoscope nor the reflex hammer was yet in use. Moreover, the modern reader finds Parkinson's literary style quaint and archaic. Nevertheless, his account is remarkable for its accuracy and clarity of expression. In a few words he cut right to the heart of the matter. His opening chapter begins with the following terse yet comprehensive definition: "*Shaking Palsy (Paralysis Agitans)*: Involuntary tremulous motion, with lessened muscular power, in parts not in action and even when supported; with a propensity to bend the trunk forwards, and to pass from a walking to a running pace; the senses and intellect being uninjured."

Some of the symptoms mentioned in this definition had been described long before. Indeed, the ancient Greek–Roman physician Galen wrote of tremor of the hand at rest and distinguished it from a tremor occurring during movement. That is, Galen made a distinction between a resting tremor and an action tremor.

It is thus tempting to believe that Galen knew of Parkinson's disease, but we cannot be certain because he does not associate the tremor with the other symptoms. Similarly, the tendency "to pass from a walking to a running pace" had also been described long before Parkinson's time. Indeed, Parkinson himself referred to a description rendered by the eighteenth-century French physician Sauvages, who had termed the abnormal gait *sclerotyrbe festinans.* On reading Sauvages's account, one feels that he had very probably seen cases of Parkinson's disease. Yet since he did not mention any other symptom, we cannot be certain. Goethe, the great German poet, noted that the innkeeper in Rembrandt's sketch "The Good Samaritan" stands in a stooped posture, holding his hands before him with the thumbs opposing the fingers as if counting coins—as patients with Parkinson's disease often do (Fig. 14). Goethe commented that the artist had been so skillful that the innkeeper's hands actually appear to tremble. One wonders if Rembrandt had intended to represent a case of Parkinson's disease, by whatever name (if any) it was known in his time. It is tempting to believe that so acute an observer as the great artist undoubtedly must have seen persons with what we now call Parkinson's disease—but again we cannot be certain.

There are other hints that Parkinson's disease has been with us a very long time. However, the possibility that James Parkinson was describing a truly new disease cannot be dismissed. A major problem is that the art of medicine was not sufficiently advanced prior to James Parkinson's time to provide much light on the subject. Very few diseases were known in their entirety. Every symptom was described as an independent entity unto itself. Medical writing was replete with descriptions of symptoms but not of entire patients.

It was only toward the end of the eighteenth century that combinations of symptoms came to be recognized as expressions of specific diseases that had a beginning, a particular pattern of evolution, and a termination. It was also at that time that symptom combinations came to be explained by, or at least correlated with, anatomic changes that were found on postmortem examination. The early nineteenth century was a time when many of the diseases known today were first described, and a beginning was made at correlating the symptoms present in life with changes found on postmortem study. Many of these diseases bear the names of the early medical investigator who first described them. Thus we have from the early nineteenth century not only Parkinson's disease but also Bright's disease, Hodgkin's disease, Bell's palsy, and so on. In many cases, the names of the early describers have been dropped, and more descriptive names have been used. In a few cases, however, no satisfactory term has been found, and so the eponym (the name of the physician who first wrote about the disease) remains in common use. Thus it is with Parkinson's disease.

No satisfactory descriptive term for Parkinson's disease has been found. The original term *shaking palsy* seems too vague. Its Latin translation, *paralysis agitans,* is no better, although it may sound more "scientific" merely because it is Latin. Diseases that were first identified from postmortem studies are often designated by terms describing the essential pathologic findings. Thus we have

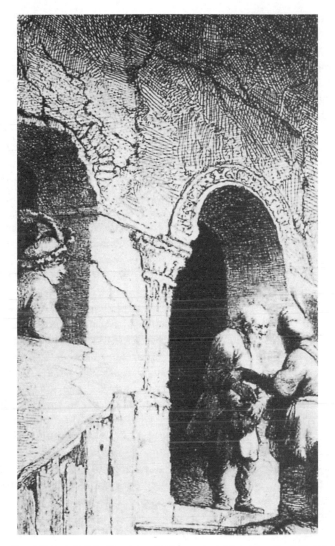

FIG. 14. The Good Samaritan in Rembrandt's famous etching. The poet Goethe thought the innkeeper had tremor of the hands. The man's appearance is suggestive of Parkinson's disease.

among nervous system disorders such entities as spinocerebellar degeneration, striatonigral degeneration (SND), and olivopontocerebellar atrophy (OPCA). These conditions are commonly known among neurologists by their acronyms, such as OPCA, because their names are otherwise too cumbersome to use. Following this pattern, we might describe Parkinson's disease as *substantia nigra atrophy.* However, Parkinson's disease was fully recognized by its signs and symptoms long before its pathology was identified, and so the name *Parkinson's disease* has been established by a long and continuous usage. There seems to be no good reason to change the name at the present time, and it seems appropriate to commemorate the history of our knowledge of the disorder in its name. After all, Parkinson deserves recognition for having connected the several symptoms he noted and for having recognized that patients at "different stages of its progress" were victims of the same disorder. This was an important contribution and a considerable accomplishment in his time.

Many other nineteenth-century physicians contributed to our knowledge of Parkinson's disease. One especially deserving mention was Jean-Martin Charcot, a great medical teacher and one of the founders of modern neurology. Charcot studied patients with the shaking palsy and considerably enlarged Parkinson's description. He added the muscular rigidity, the small handwriting (micrographia), the characteristic posturing of fingers and toes, and many other manifestations. A scholarly man with a keen interest in history, Charcot insisted that the shaking palsy should be named *Parkinson's disease* because Parkinson had been the first to describe it and the term *shaking palsy* seemed inappropriate. There was, he argued, no true paralysis or palsy (as in stroke, for example), and some patients had no tremor.

One of Charcot's students, Paul Richer, was also an artist. He is best remembered today for a textbook on human anatomy that he wrote for artists (which has recently been translated into English by Robert Hale). His sketches of Charcot's patients at the Sâlpétrière Hospital in Paris are classics of medical illustration and were widely reproduced in medical textbooks of the later nineteenth century. One of his sketches is shown in Fig. 15. The English neurologist William Gowers, one of the founders of neurology, the inventor of the ophthalmoscope and a friend of Charcot, also described the condition in great detail. He speculated about its possible cause and spoke of a loss of vitality of certain centers in the nervous system, a process he termed *abiotrophy.*

As a result of the work of Charcot, Gowers, and other medical teachers, Parkinson's disease became a well-recognized disorder by the late nineteenth century. It seems fair to say that physicians of the 1890s were as familiar with it as physicians are today.

Parkinson had been able only to speculate on the cause of the disease and on the location of the disturbance in the nervous system. He expressed the hope that "those who humanely employ postmortem anatomic examination in detecting the causes and nature of diseases" would be able to ascertain its "real nature" so that "appropriate modes of relief, or even of cure," might be found.

Many physicians engaged in studying the pathology of nervous system disorders sought to find the nature of the disease as Parkinson had hoped. Their labors, however, were for a long time unproductive, and there was much speculation regarding the site of the trouble in the brain. Some thought the problem was in the spinal cord, and others thought it was in the muscles, but no consistent abnormality could be found. Parkinson's disease was thus classified for a time as a "neurosis," meaning thereby that there was no known *structural* change

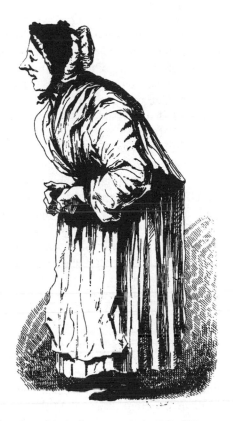

FIG. 15. Sketch of patient Anne Marie Gavr . . . . At the Sâlpétrière Hospital in Paris. Drawn by Paul Richer in 1874.

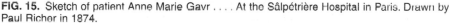

in the brain to explain the symptoms. In short, there was an obvious disturbance of function without an apparent material cause. One can readily see on reading discussions of the disease written during the 1890s that this was a perplexing and frustrating state of affairs.

One of Charcot's students, Edouard Brissaud, suggested that the material basis of Parkinson's disease might be found in a certain small nerve center, or nucleus, in the brainstem, called the *substantia nigra.* Studies of this area of the brain were later made post mortem. There was great difficulty distinguishing changes that might be due to aging, arteriosclerosis, or the disease itself. Finally, a student named Tretiakoff, working on his doctoral thesis in Paris, described a number of changes in the nerve cells of the substantia nigra that are now recognized as typical of Parkinson's disease. There was a loss of the pigmented nerve cells of this nucleus, and the spherical body first noted by Frederick Lewy was present in the remaining nerve cells. His thesis was published in 1915, nearly a century after Parkinson's *An Essay on the Shaking Palsy.* These findings were not readily accepted by the medical scientists of that time. Many neurologists were skeptical that injury to so small a group of obscure nerve cells could give rise to all the varied symptoms of parkinsonism. Others thought that loss of nerve cells in other areas, especially in the corpus striatum, was a more likely cause of the symptoms. Controversy continued on this subject for many years.

The recurrent epidemics of sleeping sickness, or encephalitis lethargica, that struck during the years from 1916 to 1926, brought great confusion to the whole subject. Rather suddenly neurologists were confronted with large numbers of relatively young patients having symptoms bearing some resemblance to those of Parkinson's disease. There were also some striking differences. The victims of this new disease were relatively young, mostly between the ages of 15 and 30, whereas, previously, parkinsonism had been extremely rare under the age 40. Suddenly the young Parkinson patient had become commonplace in the neurologic clinics and wards of big-city hospitals. These young patients had many bizarre symptoms that had never before been associated with parkinsonism.

The recognition that there could be two kinds of parkinsonism soon led to the labeling of other conditions that bore some resemblance, however remote, to Parkinson's disease as types of parkinsonism. Thus there came about the notion of arteriosclerotic parkinsonism and parkinsonism due to carbon monoxide or other chemical intoxications. The various entities became confused—so much so that during the 1930s some physicians began to suspect that all parkinsonism was due to encephalitis! A more popular view was that there was no such thing as Parkinson's disease but that "parkinsonism" was simply a fortuitous grouping of symptoms reflecting many different diseases. With the concept of parkinsonism in such a confused state, it is not surprising that pathologists had difficulty confirming Tretiakoff's findings.

The structural changes in the brain in cases of encephalitis lethargica were studied and defined. Here too the substantia nigra was consistently found to be affected. The change was thought perhaps to be related to the Parkinson symptoms; however, instead of Lewy bodies, the remaining cells contained a dense bundle of microscopic filaments called *neurofibrillary tangles.* Then a German pathologist, Dr. Rolf Hassler, studied the substantia nigra in Parkinson's disease in greater detail and confirmed the earlier findings of Tretiakoff. His work was published in 1939, but because of the disruption of World War II it received little attention for some years. After the war the noted brain pathologist Dr. J. G. Greenfield studied the brains of Parkinson patients at London's National Hospital for Nervous Diseases and further confirmed the constant involvement of the substantia nigra in Parkinson's disease. Gradually, more and more brain pathologists came to agree that here was the major site of anatomic derangement in parkinsonism and that Lewy bodies were the hallmark of Parkinson's disease, whereas neurofibrillary tangles were typical of postencephalitic parkinsonism.

The significance of the changes observed in the substantia nigra remained obscure for a long time. No one knew what the substantia nigra did or how extensive its connections were with other brain regions. Research anatomists tried to injure the substantia nigra in animals but were unable consistently to produce manifestations similar to those of human parkinsonism. There were considerable technical difficulties, and no one was quite sure how a parkinsonian cat or dog or monkey should look.

A major step forward came with the demonstration, using a new microscopic technique developed in Sweden, that the nerve cells of the substantia nigra contained the chemical substance dopamine. The new technique depended on a chemical reaction that changes dopamine into a substance that shines brightly green when placed under ultraviolet light. In the 1960s a brilliant group of young Swedish researchers, including Drs. Ungerstedt, Dahlström, Fuxe, and Anden, applied this technique to the rat brain and demonstrated whole systems of nerve cell pathways that had previously been unknown. Among these was an important system of fibers that arose from the nerve cells of the substantia nigra and went to all areas of the corpus striatum. This new discovery in the field of brain anatomy was given additional meaning by new discoveries in other areas. Biological chemists were finding that dopamine was present almost exclusively in these two regions of the brain. One researcher, Oleh Hornykiewicz, working in the medical school of the University of Vienna, measured dopamine in the brains of patients who had died with various diseases. He found a striking deficiency of dopamine in those who had parkinsonism, but not in those with other disorders. On further work he noted that the dopamine deficiency was greatest in those cases in which the pathologists found the most severe changes in the substantia nigra.

These various biochemists owed their ability to measure dopamine, adrenalin, serotonin, and related biologically active substances in brain and other tissues to the work of Dr. Julius Axelrod at the National Institutes of Health (NIH) in Bethesda, Maryland. Many of them had come to the NIH to study with Dr. Axelrod. These substances occur in minute quantities in tissue amid innumerable other similar substances. Dr. Axelrod had developed chemical techniques for separating these substances and then measuring them in extremely small samples. He thus opened an entire new field of biological chemistry. He was awarded the Nobel Prize for Physiology and Medicine in 1970 for his discovery of the enzyme, catechol-O-methyl transferase, which degrades dopamine and related chemical messengers within the nervous system after they are no longer needed to transmit nerve impulses.

Related research in animals showed that when the substantia nigra was injured, dopamine disappeared from the corpus striatum on the same side. This indicated that there must be a connection from the substantia nigra to the corpus striatum and confirmed of the existence of the *nigrostriatal* pathway. This was important because these fibers could not be demonstrated by the classic methods of brain anatomy. Brain anatomists were skeptical at first, but as this sort of evidence gradually accumulated and was confirmed by scientists in other countries, the existence of the dopamine nerve cell system gained acceptance.

In the meantime, a third key observation had been made by Professor Arvid Carlsson at the University of Göteborg in Sweden. In 1957, he carried out a simple experiment that clarified the way in which reserpine produced its tranquilizing effect. Reserpine is a major tranquilizer that can produce a condition closely resembling Parkinson's disease. Chemical measurements had shown that reserpine caused depletion of various substances in the brain, including noradrenaline, dopamine, and serotonin. Some thought that the tranquilizing effect was due to the depletion of serotonin. Professor Carlsson found that an injection of levodopa immediately reversed the tranquil state produced in the animals by reserpine, whereas the precursor of serotonin did not. He also measured the amount of dopamine in the brains of the animals and found that the levodopa had restored the dopamine levels to normal.

These discoveries achieved independently in separate scientific fields gave a new meaning to the changes in the substantia nigra first found in Parkinson patients and explained the production of parkinsonism by the tranquilizing drugs. Parkinsonism could now be defined as a state of brain dopamine insufficiency. Professors Carlsson and Hornykiewicz both suggested that levodopa might be tried as a treatment for parkinsonism. These discoveries, which so greatly clarified the nature of parkinsonism, came chiefly during the decade from 1957 to 1967. However, they represented the culmination of many decades of scientific research and thought. They could not have been achieved, say, during the 1930s or 1940s because the basic knowledge of brain chemistry was lacking. Indeed, even the fundamental techniques—such as the use of radioisotopes and the analytical techniques in organic chemistry that made possible the measurement of dopamine and related substances in the brain—were unknown before 1950. Thus it is that practical advances in medical care depend on the state of science as a whole, and that so-called pure research in basic science, with no obvious connection to practical problems, leads eventually to profound new understanding of human disease and entirely new forms of treatment.

Initially, levodopa was given in small doses by injection into a vein or in small doses by mouth. The first physicians to try levodopa were Dr. Walter Birkmayer of Vienna and Dr. Andre Barbeau of Montreal. Many others soon attempted the same approach. There was marked disagreement regarding the results. Some reported dramatic improvement even in severely affected patients. Others found no effect at all, and still others noted some minimal improvements but thought they might be due to psychological factors (such as the enthusiasm of the investigators) rather than to the levodopa effect. A thoughtful review of the evidence in 1965 indicated that the results were too limited to be of practical value for the treatment of Parkinson patients.

Then Dr. George Cotzias, a medical scientist working at the Brookhaven National Laboratories in Upton, New York, found that much larger doses by mouth yielded better results. He found that if he continued to administer dopa (at first he worked with a 50–50 mixture of D-dopa and L-dopa, or DL-dopa) every day for weeks and months, the patients gradually became tolerant of the side effects. Nausea and vomiting gradually diminished and disappeared, so that progressively larger doses could be given. By persisting patiently, raising the dose every few days as his patients slowly developed a tolerance for dopa, Dr. Cotzias was able eventually to give doses 20 to 30 times larger than the initial dose. With very large doses (as high as 12 to 18 g of DL-dopa per day), he obtained striking improvements in patients with typical and quite severe parkinsonism. The effects of dopa were clearly much greater than those attainable with the conventional anti-Parkinson drugs previously available.

Dr. Cotzias first reported his results with DL-dopa in 1967. Within a year they were confirmed at several other research centers. A large, carefully controlled study conducted by Drs. Yahr, Hoehn, Barrett, Schear, and Duvoisin at the Columbia–Presbyterian Medical Center in New York and similar studies carried out by Drs. Sweet and McDowell at New York Hospital, by Dr. Markham at the University of California in Los Angeles, and by many others helped gain acceptance of levodopa administration as a normal treatment for Parkinson's disease.

Several thousand patients were treated under research protocols at major teaching hospitals and medical research centers throughout the United States and in many other countries. Levodopa was consistently found to be more effective in the treatment of parkinsonism than any other treatment then known. The generic name *levodopa* was chosen for the medical preparation of L-dopa as a drug. It was formally approved by the Food and Drug Administration (FDA) for use in treating parkinsonism in 1970.

In the quarter century since the advent of levodopa treatment, much effort has been expended to improve its action. The dopamine receptor agonists bromocriptine (Parlodel), pergolide (Permax), pramipexole (Mirapex), and ropinirole (Requip) gradually found their place as drugs that improve the beneficial effects of levodopa. The addition of selegiline (Eldepryl) (also known generically as deprenyl) and the catechol-O-methyl transferase (COMT) inhibitors tolcapone (Tasmar) and entacapone (Comtan) provide other means of enhancing the good effects of levodopa. The demonstration that constant infusions of levodopa markedly diminish severe fluctuations of the on–off effect led to the development of slow-release, or controlled-release, formulations of levodopa in combination with carbidopa (Sinemet CR) and levodopa in combination with benserazide (Madopar HBS), which further enhance the efficacy of levodopa. These refinements and enhancements of levodopa treatment were limited but significant improvements in the treatment of parkinsonism.

THE MPTP STORY

In 1977, a young man living in Arlington, Virginia, made a fateful and unintentional discovery. An amateur chemist addicted to narcotic drugs, he satisfied his craving by synthesizing in his home laboratory a drug closely related to meperidine (Demerol, Sanofi Pharmaceuticals, Inc., New York, NY, U.S.A.). He followed a simple recipe, using easily available chemicals, outlined in a journal of medicinal chemistry. After using a hastily prepared batch of his homemade narcotic, he became acutely ill, rigid, and immobile and had to be admitted to a hospital. A physician noted the resemblance of his condition to parkinsonism and prescribed levodopa–carbidopa (Sinemet). The young man improved but had marked on–off fluctuations.

He was referred to the clinical center of the NIH. Drs. Sandford Markey, a chemist working in Dr. Irving Kopin's laboratory at the NIH, followed his recipe and studied the young man's chemical apparatus and glassware. He found that the reaction produced not only the narcotic drug the young man had desired but also a small amount of a by-product, especially if the reaction was run at too high a temperature. Analysis showed that the by-product was *N*-methylphenyl tetrahydropyridine, now widely known as MPTP.

Dr. Kopin and his colleagues found that injections of minute doses of MPTP produced a Parkinson-like condition in monkeys. An animal given even a minute dose would overnight become rigid and immobile, barely able to move very slowly, unable to eat or drink. A dose of levodopa restored the animal to normal but in an hour or so it would again become rigid and immobile, exactly as in a human patient with severe on–off fluctuations. They further found that a derivative of MPTP accumulated in the brains of these animals. On analysis the derivative proved to be a substance with the chemical name *N*-methylphenyl tetrahydropyridinium, referred to now by the acronym MPP+.

Meanwhile, the young man continued to be severely parkinsonian, responding to treatment with on–off fluctuations. Within a year he died of a narcotic overdose. His brain was studied post mortem, and it was found that the nerve cells of the substantia nigra had been totally destroyed. Dr. Stanley Burns, a neurologist also working in Dr. Kopin's laboratory, soon found that the nerve cells of the substantia nigra had also been destroyed in monkeys rendered parkinsonian by MPTP.

A description of the young man's unfortunate misadventure was published in 1979 by Dr. Glenn Davis, a young psychiatrist; Dr. Adrian Williams, a young neurologist; and others working with Dr. Kopin. It received little notice until several years later, when several drug addicts in California appeared in an emergency room with severe parkinsonism of sudden onset. They had given themselves injections of an illicit drug purchased on the street. The resemblance of this event to that of the young man from Virginia was recognized by an alert technician in the local poison control center. A neurologist called in consultation, Dr. William Langston, obtained a sample of the illicit drug from these addicts and had it analyzed. It contained MPTP!

Dr. Langston and his colleagues canvassed the local addict population and found a total of 200 who had used the same street drug. Seven of them had obvious signs of severe parkinsonism. A number were later found to have mild degrees of parkinsonism. Several other instances of MPTP-induced parkinsonism subsequently came to light. One concerned a Danish medicinal chemist who had prepared a batch of MPTP to use as a reagent in the synthesis of new analgesic drugs. He apparently allowed the MPTP to contact his skin. He became acutely ill with a flulike illness and became parkinsonian. His doctors thought he had developed postencephalitic parkinsonism. Levodopa treatment proved helpful. Years later, on learning of the toxicity of MPTP, his wife realized what had actually happened. The chemist was further studied by Dr. Kopin's group at the NIH in Bethesda, Maryland. Interestingly, there was no evidence that his parkinsonian condition had worsened over the intervening 9 years.

Dr. Langston read a paper describing the California drug addicts rendered parkinsonian by MPTP at the annual meeting of the American Academy of Neurology in San Diego, California, in April 1983. The striking resemblance of the MPTP-induced parkinsonism to Parkinson's disease naturally suggested that a similar substance occurring in nature or perhaps as a manmade environmental pollutant might be the cause of Parkinson's disease. Researchers throughout the world promptly began to study MPTP in the hope of finding the cause of Parkinson's disease.

Within a few years the mechanism of action of the drug was worked out. A key step was the finding that MPTP was converted to MPP+ by the enzyme monoamine oxidase (MAO). Drugs inhibiting that enzyme prevented the formation of MPP+. Dr. Richard Heikkila at the Robert Wood Johnson Medical School in New Brunswick, New Jersey, found that mice treated first with an inhibitor of MAO were not affected by a subsequent dose of MPTP, whereas mice receiving MPTP alone suffered destruction of the nerve cells in the substantia nigra. Drs. Langston and Ian Irwin showed the same phenomenon in monkeys.

These and other studies showed that the toxic agent was actually MPP+. MPTP was merely its precursor. Researchers then tried to determine how MPP+ worked. Dr. Solomon Snyder and his colleagues at Johns Hopkins University discovered that dopamine nerve cells avidly took up MPP+, as if it were dopamine. Drugs that blocked the uptake of dopamine into the dopamine nerve cells could also protect animals against the toxic effects of MPTP.

Drs. William Nicklas and Ivy Vyas in New Brunswick, New Jersey, soon found that, once inside the dopamine nerve cells, MPP+ acted on a small structure found in all living cells called the *mitochondrion*. All living cells contain mitochondria whose main function is to carry on the metabolism of oxygen. In a sense, the mitochondria are the lungs of the cell. Not surprisingly, they are essential to the life of the cell. Poison the mitochondria, and the cell instantly dies. The deadly fish poison rotenone is a powerful mitochondrial poison. Drs. Nicklas and Vyas found that MPP+ acted precisely as did rotenone: Both inhibit a specific enzyme system inside the mitochondria known as "complex one," thereby interrupting cellular respiration and promptly killing the nerve cells.

The discovery that MPP+ acted by poisoning the mitochondria in so highly specific a manner was met at first with skepticism, but eventually other researchers confirmed it. It then led logically to examination of the mitochondria in the brains of patients with Parkinson's disease. A group of researchers in London, including Drs. A. H. V. Schapira and John Clark (a biochemist expert on mitochondrial disorders) found that the mitochondrial enzyme affected by MPP+ and rotenone was partially deficient in the substantia nigra of patients with Parkinson's disease. Dr. Peter Jenner in London and researchers elsewhere followed up on this finding. However, it is unclear what the finding means.

The structural changes caused in the brain by MPTP have been extensively studied in animals, and it has become clear that MPTP-induced parkinsonism differs from Parkinson's disease. MPTP affects chiefly the substantia nigra. It does not affect other brain regions that are regularly affected in Parkinson's disease. Nor does it produce Lewy bodies. Our earlier hopes that MPTP might lead us to the cause of Parkinson's disease have not been realized. However, it has provided a simple, efficient way of making a laboratory animal parkinsonian and thus has been used as a tool by researchers looking for new drug treatments for parkinsonism.

The striking resemblance of MPTP-induced parkinsonism in monkeys and humans naturally suggested at first that Parkinson's disease might be due to a similar poison occurring in nature or to a man-made pollutant in our environment. Neurologists began searching for clues to some environmental factor among their patients. They looked for exposure to pesticides and clustering of Parkinson's disease cases in geographical regions. Although some reports suggested that people with the disease were more likely to have lived in rural areas than others or to have had greater exposure to agricultural chemicals, these reports have not led to any substantial breakthroughs. Comparisons of the prevalence of Parkinson's disease in different countries were attempted, but no definite clusters or major regional differences emerged. In short no clues to an environmental factor have been found.

In retrospect, we can see how the resemblance of postencephalitic parkinsonism to Parkinson's disease earlier in this century led to the search for a virus as the cause of Parkinson's disease. In the 1980s, the MPTP experience and the resemblance of MPTP-induced parkinsonism to Parkinson's disease led to a search for another kind of environmental agent, a toxin or chemical pollutant, as a possible cause. Yet we may also note that recent studies seeking evidence of exposure to environmental agents have instead found that the most important risk factor is the occurrence of Parkinson's disease in other family members. Thus, in a roundabout way, the search for the cause of Parkinson's disease has brought us to the role of heredity.

THE LEWY BODY

To the pathologist, the hallmark of Parkinson's disease visible under the microscope is a particular abnormal structure called the Lewy (pronounced la-veh) body within affected nerve cells in the substantia nigra and other areas of the brain. Lewy bodies may also be found in certain nerve cells in the spinal cord, in the sympathetic ganglia, and in the nerve cells in the walls of the esophagus and intestine! Under the microscope the Lewy body appears as a round mass about the size of a red blood cell, surrounded by a clear halo. Studied by electron microscopy, it has been found to consist of short filaments arranged randomly in a dense bundle at the center but radially like the spokes of a bicycle wheel in its outer portions. Chemical analyses using various kinds of antibodies have shown that it consists of materials called *ubiquitin* and *α-synuclein*. (Also see the discussion of genetics and α-synuclein.)

Today nearly all neurologists and neuropathologists who study parkinsonism agree: "If there are no Lewy bodies, it isn't Parkinson's disease." Put another way, what we call Parkinson's disease has come to mean that form of parkinsonism associated with Lewy bodies. Thus, when we diagnose "Parkinson's disease," we believe that Lewy bodies are present. Indeed, the pathologist's diagnosis has become more reliable than our clinical diagnosis. Some patients we thought too atypical in their symptoms to diagnose as Parkinson's disease have proven to our surprise to have the typical Lewy body changes on postmortem study. We had to conclude that despite their atypical manifestations, they really had Parkinson's disease.

INCIDENTAL LEWY BODIES

Some years ago Dr. Lysia Forno, a neuropathologist at the Veterans Hospital in Palo Alto, California, looked for Lewy bodies on postmortem study of the brains of people who had not had any nervous system disease in life. Her purpose was to study changes in the brain associated with aging. She found Lewy bodies in 6% of the "nonparkinsonian" brains she studied! Dr. William Gibb of the National Hospital in London similarly found Lewy bodies in 5.6% of nonparkinsonians more than 40 years of age and in more than 11% of those more than 80 years of age! Both Drs. Forno and Gibb found these Lewy bodies in the same places they occur in patients who had symptoms of Parkinson's disease in life; the Lewy bodies were also associated with other signs of nerve cell damage in the same areas. Thus both investigators concluded that these bodies were not merely "incidental" but that those who had these bodies in fact had Parkinson's disease that had not produced recognizable symptoms. Had these persons lived longer, they would eventually have developed Parkinson symptoms. The numbers found by Drs. Forno and Gibb tell us that there are many more people with presymptomatic Parkinson's disease than there are people who have Parkinson's disease with symptoms, perhaps ten to 15 times as many!

Postmortem studies of the brains of Parkinson patients have steadily progressed over the past quarter century. The pattern of distribution of the Lewy bodies throughout the nervous system has been extensively studied. Some 20 years ago they began to be found in the cerebral cortex as well as in the substantia nigra of some patients studied post mortem. Such patients were said to have "diffuse Lewy body disease" (see Chapter 1). Usually, such patients had symptoms of parkinsonism plus symptoms similar to those of Alzheimer's disease. Some, however, may have had only symptoms of the latter.

For a time, diffuse Lewy body disease was thought to be a separate disorder. But neuropathologists studying parkinsonian brains postmortem have been finding Lewy bodies more and more frequently in the cerebral cortex. They also find them in many other regions of the nervous system, even in the spinal cord, in nerve cell plexuses nearly everywhere—including the nerve cell plexuses in the walls of the intestine and esophagus.

Dr. Kosaka, working at the University of Yokohama, Japan, proposed that there was a spectrum of Lewy body disease and identified three groups of cases: types A, B, and C. Type A cases had many Lewy bodies throughout the brain. Type C had Lewy bodies only in the substantia nigra and other brainstem nerve centers. These cases corresponded to typical Parkinson's disease. Type B was intermediate. In a series of studies of brain specimens collected by the Parkinson's Disease Society of the United Kingdom, Drs. William Gibb, Robert Hughes, and Andrew Lees found Lewy bodies in the cerebral cortex in all cases of Parkinson's disease. They were found especially in certain regions of the brain, chiefly in the temporal lobes and in a portion of the temporal lob called the hippocampus. Now pathologists regularly find Lewy bodies in the gray matter of the cerebral hemispheres in all Parkinson patients studied post mortem. Some specimens show only a few Lewy bodies in the cerebral cortex; others show many, and all degrees in between can be found.

Dr. Margery Mark at the Robert Wood Johnson Medical School in New Brunswick, New Jersey, and Dr. Dennis Dickson, a neuropathologist at Albert Einstein Medical College in New York, have shown that the whole spectrum can be found within one family! They have thus confirmed that Kosaka's types A, B, and C are variations of the same condition.

HEREDITY

The role of heredity in Parkinson's disease has received increasing attention over the past 5 years. The notion that heredity plays a role in Parkinson's disease is not new. It was first advanced more than a century ago by William Gowers, the English neurologist we mentioned earlier. Many reports of families with several cases of parkinsonism were recorded in medical journals in the late nineteenth and early twentieth centuries. A half century ago, a young psychiatrist, Dr. Henry Mjönes, carried out a genetic study of Parkinson's disease. He was working for an advanced degree in medicine at the University of Lund, Sweden, under the supervision of Professor Sjogren, a leading geneticist of the time. A pioneering effort, it was the first systematic genetic study of Parkinson's disease.

Dr. Mjönes identified 194 patients with definite Parkinson's disease confirmed on his examination or by examinations by other physicians recorded in medical charts. He then set out to examine all the living relatives and to look up the records of deceased relatives. He found many affected brothers, sisters, and parents and identified nine families in which the condition had occurred in two or more generations. He concluded that Parkinson's disease was a hereditary disorder, probably due to a single gene mutation, transmitted from generation to generation to both men and women.

In his analysis Mjönes pointed out that the late age of onset of Parkinson's disease in many patients concealed its familial pattern. Since many patients do not develop symptoms of parkinsonism until their 70s or 80s, or sometimes even in their 90s—that is, at ages exceeding the average life span—he argued that some who carry the gene and are thus at risk for parkinsonism would not live long enough to exhibit its symptoms. Comparing the age of onset in his patients with actuarial tables of life expectancy, he calculated that only 60% of those who carry the presumed gene mutation would develop overt signs and symptoms of the disease. He also observed that some relatives had only one or two symptoms (e.g., tremor alone or tremor plus loss of facial expression). These relatives with partial parkinsonism would not ordinarily be diagnosed as having Parkinson's disease by a physician.

Mjönes argued that since they were related to a typical patient, they too had the disease and he counted them as affected. The most common of these partial manifestations was the relative who had only tremor. Mjönes's report aroused little interest at the time, and his conclusions were largely ignored. Most physicians then believed that parkinsonism was not a particular disease but merely a combination of symptoms due to many different conditions, including arteriosclerosis, encephalitis, and a variety of degenerative disorders that would someday be identified. Many believed that an environmental factor, the presumed virus responsible for encephalitis, was the cause of most cases. Mjönes was also criticized for counting the relatives with partial parkinsonism as also affected. He had no evidence to justify his doing so. Postmortem examinations of the brain had been carried out in several of his patients, but these were not helpful, for pathologists did not yet know—even in 1949—how to recognize Parkinson's disease in postmortem brain tissue samples. Dr. Mjönes was too far ahead of his time.

The late Dr. Andre Barbeau of Montreal also observed familial clustering of parkinsonism. He noted that some of his familial patients had relatives with essential tremor but interpreted this finding differently. He thought that there was a special form of parkinsonism related to essential tremor and called it *essential tremor-related parkinsonism*. More recently, Dr. David Brooks and his colleagues at the Hammersmith Hospital in London studied a number of pairs of twins and other at-risk relatives with solitary (essential) tremor, using an imaging method called positron emission tomography (PET). (See the following discussion.) The PET images almost always showed abnormal uptake of fluorodopa in a pattern typical of Parkinson's disease. This finding supports Mjönes's decision to count such individuals as secondary cases of Parkinson's disease.

Dr. Barbeau also suggested that Parkinson's disease could be the result of a combination of environment and heredity. He found that some Parkinson patients metabolized the drug debrisoquin sulfate (an antihypertensive agent) more slowly than others did. It is generally believed that these differences are genetically determined. The proportion of "slow metabolizers" of this drug was higher in a small series of Parkinson patients than in a group of normal subjects. He also noted that there seemed to be more cases of Parkinson's disease south of the St. Lawrence River than there were to the north of it, observing that the region of higher prevalence was also the region of more intense agriculture. He combined these two observations in the idea that there was an environmental toxin that was more likely to affect slow metabolizers of debrisoquin, who presumably would not be able to detoxify as efficiently as the supposedly more normal metabolizers did.

Dr. Barbeau's colleagues later withdrew the observation about slow and fast metabolizers because they found that many of the patients had taken the antihistamine diphenhydramine (Benadryl) and other drugs that influence the drug-metabolizing system. Nevertheless, the idea has continued to seem attractive. Dr. Adrian Williams and his colleagues in England have pursued this subject further and have reported other differences in liver metabolism between Parkinson patients and people without the disease.

POSITRON EMISSION TOMOGRAPHY

Positron emission tomography (PET) is a remarkable technique for imaging metabolic activities in parts of the body in three dimensions. It is a very expensive research tool requiring a large team of scientists (nuclear physicists, radio-chemists, pharmacologists, engineers, and specially trained physicians), a cyclotron, and an imaging system similar to that used in the routine CT (or CAT) scan. PET studies in the past few years have provided important insights into brain dysfunction in Parkinson's disease and have proved useful in confirming the diagnosis in borderline cases.

Essentially, PET scanning is analogous to a thyroid scan. A tracer substance, to which a radioactive atom has been attached, is administered to the subject, and the accumulation of this tracer in the organ or body part under study is monitored by radiation detectors. For example, iodine is extracted from the bloodstream by the thyroid gland with such high efficiency that virtually all the iodine is concentrated in the thyroid gland. By administering a minute amount of radioactive iodine and then placing detectors over the thyroid gland to record, one can obtain an image of the gland and identify abnormalities that cannot be detected by other methods.

To assess brain dopamine systems using PET scanning, a minute amount of levodopa to which a radioactive atom of fluorine has been attached is injected into the bloodstream. This fluorinated levodopa, or fluorodopa, travels through the body and is taken up by brain dopamine nerve cells just as if it were levodopa. There it is converted to fluorodopamine in just the same way that levodopa is converted to dopamine.

The radioactive atom (fluorine 18) used in PET emits positrons as it undergoes radioactive decay. A positron is an elemental particle equal in mass to an electron but carrying a positive electrical charge, whereas electrons are negatively charged. It is extremely short-lived and travels only a few millimeters at most before colliding with an electron. Both are annihilated on impact, releasing a brief burst of x-radiation consisting of two beams of x-rays going off in exactly opposite directions. This fact makes it possible to determine precisely where the collision occurred.

The patient having PET scanning is placed within a ring of radiation detectors that record the pairs of x-rays traveling in opposite directions given off by positron–electron collisions. Each collision thus is "seen" by a pair of detectors at opposite points on the ring. Precisely where in the brain the collision takes place is calculated. This is accomplished by using a very sophisticated system of electronic circuits linked to a powerful computer and determining the small differences in the times at which the burst of x-rays arrives at the detectors and the precise location of the detectors relative to the patient's head. From the millions of collisions taking place, the computer can make an image of the brain in much the same way that computed tomography does. The CT scanner also uses an array of detectors arranged in a series of rings. In both PET and CT scanning, these rings form a tunnel in which the patient is placed during the study.

Since fluorodopa is concentrated very rapidly within the corpus striatum, where most of the dopamine nerve fibers are located, the PET scanner "sees" an outline of the corpus striatum. Knowing the amount of fluorodopa injected and noting the intensity of the radiation arising in the corpus striatum, one can calculate the relative amount of levodopa-uptake capacity and dopamine-storage capacity in the corpus striatum. This provides a measure of the condition of the dopamine nerve cell system. Unfortunately, PET gives only a crude image, which is not sufficiently detailed to show the substantia nigra itself, where the dopamine nerve cell bodies reside.

Fluorodopa PET scanning for imaging brain dopamine systems has been used for nearly a decade now at PET centers. Decreased capacity to take up l-dopa and form dopamine in the striatum has been shown in Parkinson patients. Impairment of brain dopamine systems has been seen even before any symptoms appeared. For example, Dr. Donald Calne and his colleagues at the Tri-University PET Centre at the University of British Columbia found evidence of severely impaired brain dopamine systems in some of Dr. Langston's drug-addicted patients exposed to MPTP, even though they had no symptoms of parkinsonism. Fluorodopa PET scanning has also proved useful in presymptomatic detection of Parkinson's disease in individuals known to be at risk for the disease—at least for research purposes. Because of its expense and limited availability, PET has been limited to research use.

Dr. Kenneth Marik, at the Yale University School of Medicine, is developing a new imaging compound that is specific for dopamine cells but that can be used in an ordinary brain scanner. This should make good imaging less expensive than PET scans and more widely available.

15

Genetics: A Family Condition?

Most of us know the parents or grandparents we come from, but we go back and back, forever; we go back all of us to the very beginning; in our blood and bone and brain we carry the memories of thousands of beings....

V. S. Naipaul (A Way in the World)

That the cause of Parkinson's disease may lie within ourselves and be part of our genetic inheritance transmitted to us down the millennia through countless generations is an awesome thought to contemplate. The very idea that it may be due to a minor defect in our DNA, an error in our genetic code, that may be even more ancient than our own species *Homo sapiens,* strikes at the very depth of our sense of being. It may take time and patience to come to terms with so breathtaking an idea, but as a result of advances in the genetics of Parkinson's disease achieved in the past decade, it has become clear that genes play a major role in its cause. The implications are profound. The most important is that for the first time in history, we hold the keys that can unlock the mysteries of the basic mechanisms underlying this and related inherited diseases and thereby find methods of arresting, preventing, and even curing them.

The occasional occurrence of Parkinson's disease in familial clusters has been known for more than a century. The English neurologist William Gowers found it among his own patients in the late nineteenth century. But until recently, familial parkinsonism received little attention. Today we recognize that the condition is commonly familial. Numerous family studies have documented the pattern of inheritance. The disease in some multicase families has been mapped to specific DNA regions, and several gene mutations have already been identified. Specific gene mutations have also been identified in various conditions that often mimic Parkinson's disease, including dopa-responsive dystonia, juvenile-onset parkinsonism, spinocerebellar atrophy, multiple system atrophy, and the recently recognized frontotemporal dementia. Evidence for a genetic mechanism has also been found in progressive supranuclear palsy and in the related condition given the unwieldy name of *corticobasal degeneration.* These are all conditions that often masquerade as Parkinson's disease, at least in their early stages, and that can challenge the diagnostic skills of the ablest neurologists. In a clear harbinger of the future, DNA testing has already been used successfully to distinguish some of these conditions from each other and from Parkinson's disease.

FAMILIAL PARKINSON'S DISEASE

In contemporary medical usage, we say a patient is a "familial" case if he or she reports that one or more blood relatives—whether a brother, sister, parent or grandparent—are or were affected by the same condition. This information does not necessarily mean that a condition is hereditary or genetic because infections or poisons can sometimes affect multiple members of a family, though usually at about the same time. However, familial disorders are mostly inherited. The two words have often been combined into the expression *heredofamilial* to indicate a condition believed to be truly hereditary or genetic in origin. A report of secondary cases in the family needs to be confirmed by further inquiry before one concludes that the condition is indeed familial. Sometimes reported secondary cases turn out to have a different condition. Of course, the opposite may also occur. For example, an older affected family member may be said to have had a stroke but on examination turn out to have Parkinson's disease.

Estimates of the proportion of Parkinson's disease patients who are familial have varied over the past century or so from 10% to 20%. These numbers were based on retrospective reviews of medical records. Information about affected relatives was not, however, collected in a systematic way and mostly reflected the patients' responses when asked on their initial interview in a clinic or physician's office if anyone else in their family had the same condition. Nor were the reportedly affected relatives examined to confirm the report. Thus these numbers are only rough estimates. Nonetheless, they are consistent with some role for heredity.

In speaking to patient support groups throughout the United States and Canada, we have for many years asked the patients in our audiences who had affected relatives to raise their hands. Invariably, about a one-fourth to one-third of the patients have raised their hands in affirmative response. Mostly, they described small family clusters of two or three affected people, usually in two generations. Occasionally, some reported they had affected relatives in several preceding generations in their families. At first, we were skeptical of these responses, but when so many patients in so many different communities across the land so consistently gave us the same response, we realized we had to look into the familial patterns of parkinsonism more seriously. We also had become increasingly aware with the passage of years that some of our new patients were the children or younger siblings of patients we had seen a decade or two earlier. We could not simply dismiss these patients' concerns and tell them their condition was not familial. They wanted meaningful counseling on the genetic aspects of the disorder, and to provide such counseling, we needed to gain more definitive data on the subject.

To find out more precisely how frequently Parkinson's disease ran in families our geneticist, Dr. Alice Lazzarini, questioned all 216 consecutive patients whom RCD had seen in our clinic during calendar year 1991. She interviewed these patients and their families to identify all first- and second-degree relatives; that is, all brothers and sisters, both parents, all four grandparents, and all aunts and uncles. She then called upon all living relatives to find those who might be affected. We and our colleagues, Drs. Margery Mark, Lawrence Golbe, and Thomas Zimmerman, then examined those living relatives who were reported to have any parkinsonian symptoms. We traveled across the country to visit those unable to come to us. To identify deceased relatives, Dr. Lazzarini obtained birth, marriage, and death certificates in various public registries and tracked down old medical records, including old autopsy records.

On analyzing the resulting data, Dr. Lazzarini found that 26% of the patients had at least one affected relative. Most had no known affected relatives. However, *known* is a key word here, for she also found that most patients had little or no information on the fates of their grandparents or their aunts and uncles. In only 23% of the patients could reliable information be obtained on all first- and second-degree relatives. It may seem surprising at first that so few patients could give a full account of their families. We challenge you, the reader, to jot down your own family tree and see how well you can do.

Chances are you will find, perhaps to your surprise, that you did not know all four of your grandparents. Some may have died before you were born or when you were a small child. You probably have little notion of what illnesses even those you did know may have had. You probably do not know the fates of all your aunts and uncles. Some of you may have lost one of your parents in childhood. Perhaps your parents were divorced decades ago, or your father abandoned the family when you were a child. Some of you may have lost portions of your family in the great wars of the twentieth century or in the holocaust. Finally, a small number of you may be orphans and have no knowledge at all of your parents or any forebears.

Many of our patients provided hints and suggestions that some ancestors had been affected. For example, a grandparent who had lived a full life and passed away a half century ago was remembered by the family to have had a tremor in the last few years of his or her life and may have walked leaning forward with a shuffling gait. However, no one now living knew whether a medical diagnosis of parkinsonism was ever made. Medical records in such circumstances are rarely available. The ancestor in question may well have had Parkinson's disease, but we could not be certain and so could not count that person as a secondary case. In some cases, symptoms of parkinsonism may have been obscured by another disorder, such as Alzheimer's disease, strokes, or severe arthritis.

To complicate matters further some affected relatives deliberately concealed their illness from the rest of the family. An example is an elderly patient who reported that his brother had tremor of the hands and that he never visited him because he did not want his brother to know of his own affliction. Nor would he permit us to visit other living relatives. Thus there were some secondary cases we were unable to include in our study.

When Dr. Lazzarini's analysis considered only those patients for whom we were able to obtain information on both parents, all brothers and sisters, all four grandparents and all aunts and uncles, the proportion with one or more definitely affected relatives rose to about 50%. Surprisingly, large as this number is, for several reasons we believe the true proportion of patients who are truly familial is even greater! One reason is that our study was a "snapshot" of a single moment in time. Were the study of the same patients repeated after an interval of, say, 5 or 10 years, the proportion would rise as the patients' relatives aged and more of them became affected. Another reason is that at least some of the relatives we classified as possibly affected would have developed more manifestations after a few years and been reclassified as definitely affected. Still another reason is that because of the late age at which Parkinson symptoms may first appear, it is likely that some of the reportedly unaffected deceased relatives, even those who died in their 70s and 80s, would have developed signs and symptoms of the disease had they lived longer. In a survey of the population of Glasgow, Scotland, done in the 1980s, Dr. William Mutch and his colleagues found that the median age of onset of Parkinson's disease was in the mid-70s. That means that for half of all the patients they found, the onset of the disease occurred after 75 years of age. We have seen onset of the disease in the 90s, and even after 100 years of age! Thus a study such as Dr. Lazzarini carried out cannot avoid underestimating the full role of heredity.

SPORADIC PARKINSON'S DISEASE?

We are still left with a large number of patients who seem to have no affected relatives. In contemporary medical practice such patients are said to be "sporadic" cases. What does that mean? Physicians often speak of "sporadic" versus "familial" cases, with the implication that these are somehow different. But *sporadic* may only mean that, for the various reasons we have already discussed, the patient has insufficient knowledge of his or her family tree. Moreover, we have repeatedly noticed over the years that patients thought initially to be sporadic have turned out later— often many years later—to be familial when symptoms developed in a parent, brother, or sister, or when more information was discovered about their family trees. An example is provided by a retired teacher with Parkinson's disease whose mother developed parkinsonism in her 80s, 15 years after he began to have his symptoms! Another patient thought he was the only family member affected when we first saw him. Ten years later, he discovered at a family reunion that a sister he had not seen in many years also had Parkinson's disease. Although he had corresponded with her all those years, his sister had never told him that she was also affected.

Thus one can never be certain that a "sporadic" case is truly sporadic. Moreover, sporadic and familial cases do not differ in their symptoms, findings on physical examination, or results on any diagnostic tests. We have therefore concluded that the sporadic and familial cases do not represent different types of parkinsonism and that the term *sporadic* does not indicate a different cause or mechanism of disease. It simply means that there is no knowledge of affected relatives at this time.

THE PATTERN OF INHERITANCE

When our patients had two or more affected relatives, we found that nearly all occurred on the same side of the family. For example, if a patient's father had the disease, then all other affected relatives in the family were paternal relatives. This pattern has been found in a number of other studies. It is the pattern one expects in an inherited condition. In contrast, in diseases caused by environmental toxins or infectious agents, affected family members occur equally among both sides of the family.

Dr. Lazzarini and our colleague Dr. Richard Myers of Boston University further analyzed our data to calculate the lifetime risk of developing Parkinson's disease for the relatives of 80 of our familial cases. They found the risk to be 42% for the siblings of our patients and 45% for the parents. This is close to the 50% risk one would theoretically expect in a dominantly inherited disorder in conformity with Mendel's laws of heredity. Very similar results have been reported by other genetic studies of Parkinson's disease in other countries.

These data provide powerful evidence that Parkinson's disease is transmitted in a pattern geneticists call *autosomal dominant*. To explain these two terms, we need to briefly review some elements of genetics. DNA, the chemical stuff of inheritance, is distributed among a group of structures called chromosomes present in the nucleus of every cell in our bodies. They are called *chromosomes* (from the Greek, meaning "colored bodies") because they take the color of certain chemical stains that render them visible under a microscope. Chromosomes come in pairs, one received from each parent. Two of the chromosomes, named "X" and "Y," are the sex chromosomes. Males have both an X chromosome inherited from their mothers and a Y chromosome inherited from their fathers. Females have two X chromosomes, one inherited from each parent. The remaining 22 pairs of chromosomes are called *autosomes*. We can infer that gene mutations giving rise to Parkinson's disease cannot be located on the sex chromosomes since the disease occurs with equal frequency in men and women. They must therefore be on one or another autosome. Hence, Parkinson's disease is an autosomal disorder.

The term *dominant* indicates that a single copy of the causative gene mutation suffices to cause the disease. In contrast, there are also recessive disorders such as cystic fibrosis or the muscular dystrophies. In autosomal recessive inheritance, symptoms of the disorder do not develop in individuals carrying a single copy of the disease gene inherited from one parent plus a normal copy inherited from the other parent. Such individuals are carriers because they can transmit the gene mutation to their progeny. Symptoms of recessive disorders develop only in those who receive two copies of the disease gene, one from each parent. That can only occur if both parents are carriers of the disease gene.

As might be expected from these facts, each offspring of an affected person with a dominant disorder has a 50% chance of inheriting the disease gene. Moreover, the disease will regularly appear in successive generations. In contrast, offspring of parents who are both carriers of a recessive disease gene have each only a 25% chance of inheriting the disease genes of both parents and thus of being at risk to develop the disease. Since carriers of a recessive disorder do not themselves develop symptoms of the disease, it is apparent that the disease may skip generations and will appear infrequently in an affected family tree. Most recessive disorders manifest themselves in infancy or childhood.

Although each offspring of a parent afflicted with a dominant disorder has a 50% chance of inheriting the disease gene mutation, some of those actually inheriting the disease gene may for various reasons fail to develop symptoms of the disease during their lifetime. Geneticists express this fact by speaking of incomplete or partial penetrance. In the case of Parkinson's disease, an obvious reason for incomplete penetrance is the late age of onset of the symptoms. Many patients do not develop symptoms of Parkinson's disease until their 80s or 90s, beyond the average human lifespan. Estimates of penetrance for the disease vary from 60% to 80%.

The penetrance of Parkinson's disease is thus not only partial but also linked to age; it is "age-related." Just as the disease is rare among those under 40 years of age and more common among the elderly, its penetrance is also very low among those below the age of 40 years and greater among the elderly.

LARGE, MULTICASE FAMILIES

We owe much of what we know about the familial nature of Parkinson's disease and its pattern of inheritance to the study of families in which many members have been affected in several successive generations. Large families also greatly facilitate the search for underlying causative gene mutations. Let us review here several of the families in which postmortem examination of the brain has confirmed the diagnosis. It is very important to have postmortem confirmation to make sure we are dealing with true Parkinson's disease and not other disorders whose symptoms may mimic those of Parkinson's disease.

The Contursi Kindred

Our associate Dr. Lawrence Golbe discovered among our patients an especially large family, comprising several hundred people, in which 60 individuals were known to have had Parkinson's disease. All the affected individuals were descendants of a couple born in the village of Contursi in the province of Salerno in southern Italy about 1700. Not surprisingly, medical information was available only for the last six of the 12 known generations. Several members of the family immigrated to the United States between 1900 and 1920. Some descendants of both the immigrants and those who remained in Italy developed Parkinson's disease. In a collaborative project, Professors Giuseppe Di Iorio and Vincenza Bonavita of the Neurology Faculty at the University of Naples in Italy studied the Italian branches of the family while Dr. Golbe studied the American branches. About half of the patients lived all their lives in Italy; the other half lived in the United States, mainly in New York City and adjacent areas. An affected member of the family had consulted one of us (RCD) in 1965 and another member of the family had consulted RCD in 1980. Still another was a patient of JS. Postmortem confirmation of the diagnosis was made in two cases. Lewy bodies were present in the appropriate places, leaving no doubt that the family disease was true Parkinson's disease.

This was the first multicase family in which we could be certain that the disease was truly Parkinson's disease and not merely a form of parkinsonism. It was sufficiently large to permit detailed genetic analysis. The pattern of inheritance was clearly autosomal dominant. Men and women were equally likely to develop the disease. Forty percent of the family members aged 50 years or more were affected. The age of onset varied from 20 years to 85 years; the mean or average age of symptom onset was 46. There were no differences in the signs and symptoms, response to treatment, or any other particulars between the disease in the Italian and American branches of this family. This argues against a role for environmental factors in this family.

The Iowa Kindred

Subsequently, a considerable number of similar families, most with postmortem confirmation of the diagnosis, were identified in the United States, Europe, and Japan. One of the best studied of these families with information covering several generations was a kindred followed at the Mayo Clinic in Rochester, Minnesota, since 1920. The family was followed by several successive generations of Mayo Clinic neurologists, most recently by Drs. Manfred Muenter and Demetrios Maraganore, who published a detailed report of the family in 1998. A total of 22 people were affected; however, several family members had only mild tremor of the hands, which led Drs. Muenter and Maraganore to wonder whether they had essential tremor or were formes frustes (partial presentation) of the family disease! Postmortem examinations carried out at the Mayo Clinic in several affected members leave no doubt that this family suffered from Parkinson's disease.

A family encountered in southern California by Dr. Cheryl Waters of the University of Southern California, also with postmortem confirmation of the diagnosis, was later found to be a branch of the Iowa family.

Other Families

Six large American families were found in the Midwest by Dr. Zbigniew Wzollek. The families were descendants of immigrants from Germany and Denmark. Postmortem confirmation was obtained in several of these families. Dr. Golbe studied a family from Pennsylvania in which seven people were affected in four generations. Postmortem confirmation of typical Parkinson's disease was obtained in one family member.

These families, and many others like them too numerous to describe here, confirm that true Parkinson's disease does occur as a hereditary condition. The pattern of inheritance in all these families is consistently that of an autosomal dominant disorder. A single gene mutation in each family would be sufficient to cause the disease. The fact that the symptoms are similar in different branches of the same family living in different parts of the world argues against a role for environmental factors.

FORMES FRUSTES

We have found in our studies of families that some relatives have very mild symptoms for many years. They have an incompletely developed parkinsonism. Physicians call such cases *formes frustes,* from the French, meaning a "condition whose development has been frustrated." These individuals with one or two mild symptoms had not sought medical attention. If they had, they were not diagnosed as having Parkinson's disease. Some with only tremor as a symptom may be diagnosed with essential tremor. An example is a man who had the onset of tremor of the right hand at 25 years of age. When seen at age 82, he still had only tremor of the right hand! A physician himself, he believed that he had essential tremor, although he knew that his younger brother had Parkinson's disease and that essential tremor almost invariably affects both sides of the body. However, on examination he had a number of telltale signs of Parkinson's disease, including a mild rigidity of the muscles of the right arm and loss of the normal swing of that arm on walking. His tremor was also present at rest and had a typical pill-rolling character, which does not happen in essential tremor. There can be little question that his correct diagnosis was Parkinson's disease.

GENE MUTATIONS

Multiple-case families make it possible for modern molecular DNA analysis to pinpoint the location of a gene mutation and to find the mutation itself. The descriptions of so many multicase families in the 1990s aroused the interest of geneticists in research centers both in the United States and abroad. Large multi-disciplinary teams of neurologists, clinical geneticists, molecular geneticists, and scientists in related fields began to search for linkage of the disease with specific DNA sequences or "markers" in multicase families. Within a very short time, a research team led by Drs. William Nussbaum and Mihael Polymeropoulos at the National Human Genome Center, the National Institutes of Health in Bethesda, Maryland, linked the Contursi family disease to a small region of chromosome 4 in 1996. In the following year, they identified the gene and the specific mutation involved. It has been called the *Park I gene*. It turned out to be a previously known gene, which codes for a protein of unknown function named *α-synuclein*. The mutation consisted of the deletion of a single nucleotide from the DNA sequence. This resulted in the deletion of a single amino acid from that protein!

DNA consists of chains of four molecules known as nucleotides arranged in specific sequences. These chemical units—represented by the letters *A, C, G ,* and *T*—in essence are the letters of the genetic code. Each group of three nucleotides specifies a particular amino acid in the construction of a protein. In this manner, the coding region of a gene determines the amino acids and the sequence in which they are linked in a chain to make a protein. The total sequence of some 1 billion nucleotides in the human genome spells out the instructions for building an entire human being. Tiny variations in the code make each of us, except for identical twins, unique individuals. There are a great many variations due to the replacement of a single nucleotide by another. These are known as *single nucleotide polymorphisms,* or SNPs. Most of these variations are of unknown significance and are believed to be harmless. However, some SNPs, as in the Contursi family, determine an individual's risk for particular diseases.

We were disappointed that extensive searches through hundreds of families in many research centers found the Contursi mutation in only a handful of other families. It turned out to be a very rare cause of Parkinson's disease. Curiously, except for the Contursi kindred, it has been found so far only in a few families of Greek origin deriving from a small region of western Greece. We speculate that the Contursi family may have descended from Greek families who immigrated to southern Italy centuries ago, for we know that there has been close contact between the two regions since ancient times.

A second mutation in the gene for α-synuclein was discovered in a German family by Dr. R. Kruger of Ruhr-University in Bochum, Germany. It is also an SNP. So far, it has not been found in any other family and thus also appears to be a very rare cause of Parkinson's disease. It is possible that additional mutations in this gene may be found. A team led by Dr. John Hardy of the Mayo Clinic, Jacksonville, Florida, linked the Iowa family described earlier to a region of chromosome 4 distant from the gene for α-synuclein. A team of geneticists led by Dr. Thomas Gasser of the University of Munich, Germany, has linked the disease in the German-American families collected by Dr. Wzollek to a small region of chromosome 2. Specific genes have not yet been identified in these families.

A specific mutation in the gene for a protein named *unbiquitin carboxy-terminal hydrolase* was found in another German family. The protein is an enzyme, which helps cells dispose of damaged proteins. It is not known what protein it normally works on, but its activity is greatly reduced by the mutation. Again, this mutation was not found in other patients, and so, like the α-synuclein mutations, it is a rare cause of Parkinson's disease.

In summary, the several gene mutations and DNA loci so far linked to Parkinson's disease can account for only a tiny percentage, probably less than 1%, of all cases of the disease. Thus right from the outset the genetics of the disease has proved to be unexpectedly complex. We had hoped that, as in the case of many other inherited diseases, a single mutation might have accounted for all Parkinson's disease, but this hope was not realized. Instead, we face the prospect of many different genes linked to Parkinson's disease, each probably subject to a number of mutations. How many is anybody's guess at this time.

There is some suggestion that the disease varies somewhat in the different families, although there is enormous variation within each family. For example, the average age of onset is lower in the Contursi kindred than in the German-American families collected by Dr. Wzollek, and it is lower still in the Iowa kindred. Thus we may find that each gene mutation causes a somewhat unique disease. Instead of one Parkinson's disease, we may find that there are many. However, because of the large variations within each family and a great deal of overlap between families, it will not be possible to guess which mutation is at hand in a particular patient from the signs and symptoms or any laboratory tests other, of course, than DNA testing.

α-Synuclein

The discovery that a mutation in the gene coding for the protein α-synuclein causes Parkinson's disease has aroused widespread interest in that protein among scientists in diverse fields. They have begun to study the normal function of this protein, to search for the abnormalities occurring in the protein as a result of the mutation, and to investigate how abnormalities in this protein may cause disease. The first surprise was that the Lewy body (see Chapter 1), that abnormal body found in the degenerating nerve cells in the substantia nigra and other regions in Parkinson's disease, is filled with α-synuclein. Indeed, demonstrating the presence of this protein in the affected nerve cells by antibody techniques has proved superior to other methods of demonstrating Lewy bodies. It has become the new standard for the diagnosis of Parkinson's disease in brain tissue samples.

An important point is that α-synuclein accumulation was found in the brain in all cases of Parkinson's disease, not only in those with the Contursi mutation. Moreover, it accumulates in abnormal amounts in the nerve cells of the substantia nigra and in the many other nuclei as well in the areas of cerebral cortex affected in Parkinson's disease. Thus it appears that some abnormality of α-synuclein is common in all cases of Parkinson's disease and relates in some way to the basic mechanism of the disease.

JUVENILE-ONSET PARKINSONISM

For several decades, Japanese neurologists have described a form of parkinsonism initially thought to be unique to Japan. It differed from "typical" Parkinson's disease in having a younger age of onset. Indeed, the Japanese neurologists named it *juvenile-onset parkinsonism,* by which they meant onset before the age of 40 years. Dystonia was also more severe and frequent than in "typical" Parkinson's disease. Finally, it differed from Parkinson's disease in a crucial particular. The anatomic changes in the brain on postmortem study were different. There were no Lewy bodies! The disorder also differs from Parkinson's disease in that it is inherited in an autosomal recessive manner. Parkinson's disease, in contrast, is an autosomal dominant disorder.

Japanese neurologists and geneticists led by Dr. Mizuno of Juntendo University in Tokyo linked the disorder to a region of chromosome 6. They subsequently identified the gene involved and named it the *Parkin gene*. They found a variety of mutations in the gene in different families, all consisting of deletions from the gene of various DNA segments, some larger and some very small. The normal function of the protein encoded by the Parkin gene is not yet known.

As often happens when a disorder is first discovered in one population group, it soon is found in others. Patients with this form of parkinsonism due to deletions in the Parkin gene have now been found in Europe, North Africa, the Middle East, and the United States. Some have disease onset later in life than in the cases that were first recognized. Some appear to be sporadic, which probably reflects the greater difficulty of identifying secondary cases in recessively inherited disorders. Moreover, despite the important differences from Parkinson's disease, in individual cases it may be difficult to distinguish the two conditions from analysis of the symptoms and the findings of the physical examination. It is clear that some patients now diagnosed as having Parkinson's disease in fact have the Parkin gene disorder. Our colleague, Dr. Lawrence Golbe, had treated a member of such a family in our clinic. He had thought it was just another case of Parkinson's disease until DNA testing done as part of a research program revealed that the family harbored the Parkin gene!

While such testing is presently available only on a research basis, this experience shows how DNA testing may be used to identify which type of parkinsonism a patient may have. It also suggests that when DNA testing of Parkinson's disease patients becomes more generally available, we may find that cases due to the Parkin gene deletions are not uncommon.

A FAMILY DISEASE

As we come to terms with the fact that heredity plays a large role in Parkinson's disease, the patient is no longer the sole subject of attention. The entire family deserves consideration. A host of new questions arise. What are the chances that other family members may become affected? When? What should I tell my family? Can the disease skip a generation? Can those at risk be identified through presymptomatic DNA testing? If so, should they be tested? Can the disease be prevented in those who test positive? In short, genetic counseling is becoming part of the medical management of parkinsonism.

Unfortunately, our ability to answer these questions is at present rather limited. Only in the rare families in which the gene is known is it possible to do presymptomatic DNA testing, but at present this can only be done in a research setting. In current research protocols, the test results are not shared with the subjects of the research because of the potential for great emotional distress. Learning that one has tested negative for the gene mutation may be very reassuring. However, learning that one has tested positive and is thus likely to develop the disease at some unknown future date can be quite traumatic, especially since as yet we have no means of preventing the disease or of arresting its course.

All we can do at present for the average Parkinson's disease patient who is not a member of a family in which the underlying gene mutations is known is to make a rough estimate of the risk of parkinsonism developing within a normal lifetime in an offspring of an affected parent. Some years ago, Dr. Leonard Kurland, a neurologist and epidemiologist at the Mayo Clinic, estimated the lifetime risk of Parkinson's disease developing in any individual to be 2.5%, or one in 40. Clearly, the risk to the children of an affected parent will be somewhat greater than that. The observed prevalence of secondary cases of Parkinson's disease among relatives is about 6% to 7%, or roughly three times the rate in the general population. Genetic counselors thus quote a threefold greater lifetime risk for unaffected relatives as compared with the general population risk, but this is little more than a cautious guess. Recent analyses of multicase families indicate that for an individual with an affected parent and brother or sister, the lifetime risk averages about 25%. In families with several known secondary cases in two or more generations, it is possible to make a more precise estimate of the risk. Obviously, it may be higher in families in which the average age of onset is lower than in other families in which the age of onset is higher. The risks may depend on which gene mutation affects a particular family.

As we stated earlier, Parkinson's disease is an autosomal dominant disorder and 50% of the offspring of affected parents will, on average, harbor the causative gene mutation. But as we mentioned in our discussion of penetrance, not all those who have the gene mutation will develop symptoms of the disease in a normal lifetime. So the lifetime risk will be less than 50%. When we consider that half the patients in the general population have their symptom onset after 75 years of age, we come to the conclusion that the risk is probably not more than 25% to 30%. Moreover, we know that many secondary cases are formes frustes with very minimal symptoms. Many have only mild tremor. They may not have enough symptoms to warrant the diagnosis or require any treatment! We would thus estimate that the risk of developing the full-blown disease with all the major symptoms is less than 25%, and more likely only about 10% to 15%.

Taking all these facts and estimates into account, we conclude that, considering all the other disease and accidents that can happen over the course of a lifetime, the risk of passing Parkinson's disease on to one's offspring should not be a major source of concern. At this time, we do not recommend that unaffected relatives or offspring of a patient seek examination in the hope of finding out whether they are also affected.

16

Future Prospects

The introduction of levodopa treatment in the late 1960s resulted from important scientific advances that led to the discovery of dopamine in the brain and its deficiency in parkinsonism. That led logically to the use of levodopa to correct the deficiency, and it worked unexpectedly well. The treatment of Parkinson's disease became rational and far more effective than ever before. There have been many minor refinements and improvements in treatment since then. But all these improvements were based on dopamine deficiency. These included better means of delivering dopamine to the deprived brain regions, as well as drugs imitating the actions of dopamine, or extending or enhancing its actions.

It seems clear that another major advance in treatment can only come from another major advance in our understanding of the fundamental nature of Parkinson's disease. That is, the next major advance in treatment will come from an understanding of the basic mechanisms of the disease process itself. To put it more bluntly, to find a cure we must find the cause. We must find out why those dopamine nerve cells are sick in the first place, so that we can rationally develop means of correcting or preventing their illness. And we will also need to consider all the other nerve cell systems that are affected in the disease.

That will require a very major advance indeed in our understanding of the disease. It will come from a previously unexpected quarter and from a scientific technology that was developed only in the past decade. That is, it will come from modern molecular genetics.

GENETICS

The discovery of two mutations in the gene for the protein α-synuclein in Parkinson's disease families and the finding that Lewy bodies contain large amounts of this protein herald the beginning of a new understanding of Parkinson's disease. The question arises, "Could Parkinson's disease be due to an abnormality in the metabolism of α-synuclein?" As one might expect, scientists in disciplines such as protein chemistry and cell biology who previously had no reason to be concerned with the disease have been drawn to that question and are seeking to unravel how α-synuclein is altered in the disease and what role it may play in the disease process. There is already evidence that the known mutations in that protein cause abnormal aggregations of the protein, binding to other proteins and causing various adverse effects on nerve cell function. It is beginning to appear that α-synuclein plays a central role in the mechanism of Parkinson's disease. We may expect future research to build upon these new findings and perhaps lead to entirely new forms of treatment.

The fact that within 3 years Parkinson's disease was mapped to six different locations on the human genome signals an auspicious beginning. It also suggests, however, that the genetics of the disease will be complex and that mutations in many different genes will eventually be found capable of causing the disease. In the present state of the art of molecular genetics with the ability to perform very rapid sequencing of DNA segments, if one has a family with ten or so affected members in at least two generations, it is possible to pinpoint a DNA marker and to identity a gene rather quickly. Families of that size are relatively easy to find and document. So we would expect that within a few more years new gene mutations will be found.

The announcement in June 2000 that scientists had finished sequencing the entire human genome as well as the recent advances in the genetics of Parkinson's disease raises the hope of greatly accelerating that process. Having the entire genome available will greatly simplify the search, especially the search for single-nucleotide polymorphisms (SNPs). Geneticists will no longer need to rely only on well-documented families. Nor will they need to sequence long stretches of DNA in each new family or group of patients. Instead, they will be able to rely on the sequences already established by the human genome project. Special computer chips coated with DNA that can detect SNPs when an individual's DNA is tested against him or her will make it possible to rapidly screen large numbers of patients at random looking for associations with particular SNPs.

Competition to identify the genetic basis of Parkinson's disease and other nervous system disorders will be intense in the universities, in government laboratories, and in private industry. In the past several years, all the major pharmaceutical firms have developed departments of genetics, and their directors are often represented on their firms' governing boards. Countless smaller biotech firms have been founded to work on the genetics of human disease. They know that the future of medicine lies in genetics.

The task ahead is not a simple one. We are faced with the prospect of numerous mutations in many different genes, all capable of causing Parkinson's disease. Despite the enormous research power of modern molecular genetics and cell biology, it will take some years to identify at least a major portion of the causative gene mutations and unravel their mechanisms of action and their interactions with other genes and possibly with environmental factors. Yet it appears likely that many different gene mutations may cause abnormalities in α-synuclein and lead to the same result. One may thus speculate that various means of preventing the accumulation of α-synuclein might delay or prevent the progression of Parkinson's disease. We may expect research directed to that goal. Should such research be successful, we might for the first time have treatments that actually attack the underlying disease process itself.

To study the role of α-synuclein will require the development of animals carrying one of the gene mutations causing human Parkinson's disease. We expect that attempts will be made to transfer one of the α-synuclein mutations into the genome of such animals as the laboratory mouse. Such an animal is called a *transgenic animal.* Strains of transgenic mice carrying the mutation and passing it on to their offspring will then be available for research. Of course, it is possible that such mice will not develop Parkinson's disease even if they do develop accumulations of α-synuclein in the brain in the right places. However, if transgenic animals can be bred and they do develop Lewy bodies, then it will be possible to search for means of blocking the accumulation of α-synuclein in the affected brain cells. Transgenic mice are now used in research in other neurodegenerative disorders, such as Alzheimer's disease and amyotrophic lateral sclerosis (Lou Gehrig's disease) to give just two examples. At least in the case of Alzheimer's disease, these animals have already led to new experimental therapies. Transgenic mice could also lead to new treatments for Parkinson's disease.

STEM CELLS

There is much excitement in the scientific community over the potential of stem cells, both for research and as a source of cells for transplantation to the parkinsonian brain. Although articles in the public media often speak of such cell transplants as a "cure," this is not the case. The transplants envisaged are dopamine-producing cells derived from stem cells that could be grown in the laboratory and used to replace the degenerated dopamine-producing nerve cells of the substantia nigra. The only difference from fetal cell transplants is the source of the cells.

Stem cell–derived tissue would bypass the ethical quandaries of using human fetal brain cells for transplantation and may lower the risk of infection. These are important considerations but we should remember that transplantation represents a symptomatic treatment. It may yield significant benefit to a small number of selected patients, but it is in no sense curative. We already know that fetal cell transplants do not slow the progression of Parkinson's disease. There is no reason to believe transplants derived from stem cells would yield a different result.

The limitations of transplant therapy arise from the fact that loss of the dopamine producing cells of the substantia nigra is only one part of Parkinson's disease. Many other nerve cell systems throughout the entire nervous system are affected and other chemical messengers are also depleted including noradrenalin, acetylcholine and others not yet identified. We understand that enthusiasm for recent technical and scientific advances may lead to exaggerated hopes and claims, but we should recognize hype when we see it. While stem cells undoubtedly will lead to new understanding of nerve cell development, it is difficult to see how their use could lead to a cure for Parkinson's or any other degenerative nervous system disease.

NERVE GROWTH FACTORS

Proteins somewhat like insulin have been found to play an important role in regulating the growth of nerve cells and in maintaining them throughout life. These have been called "nerve growth factors" (NGF), or neurotrophins. One of these factors, called *sympathetic nerve growth factor,* was first discovered a half century ago by Dr. Rita Levi–Montalcini of Italy. This substance was at first thought to act only on the sympathetic nerves. Later, however, it was found to stimulate the growth of the cholinergic nerve cells in the brain, specifically those in a cluster of cells in the upper brainstem called the *nucleus basalis of Meynert.* The cells of this nucleus are affected in Alzheimer's disease, and their loss is thought to underlie the memory impairments typical of that condition. These cells are also affected in Parkinson's disease. More recently, other NGFs that act on the dopamine nerve cells of the substantia nigra have been found. Among these are "brain-derived" NGF (BDNGF) and "glial-derived" NGF (GDNGF). Both of these received much attention at first, and it was suggested that they might be used to treat Parkinson's disease.

Direct administration of NGFs has been attempted experimentally in animal models and inpatients with a variety of nervous system disorders. Administration of NGF directly into the brain has been attempted experimentally in the treatment of Alzheimer's disease, but the results are not satisfactory. Another factor, called *ciliary growth factor,* has been tried in amyotrophic lateral sclerosis (Lou Gehrig's disease)—again without definite benefit. In fact, it appeared to make some cases worse. An NGF has also been tried in diabetics with peripheral nerve involvement. The results of a trial of GDNGF in Parkinson patients were disappointing.

Because these factors are proteins, they can reach their target nerve cells only if injected directly into the brain. They do not spread through the brain, so they must be injected very near the target nerve cells. Thus researchers are turning to indirect methods of inducing the brain to produce more such factors. Unfortunately, the nerve growth factors have turned out to be far more complicated than had initially been suspected. There are entire families and subfamilies of these factors. Each type of nerve cell and each nucleus of brain cells appear to have its own specific family of such factors, yet these factors act at many different sites. In view of the multiplicity of NGFs and the complexity of their actions, neuroscientists will need to learn a great deal more about them. We can only speculate at this time whether manipulation of NGFs may lead to new therapeutic approaches to Parkinson's disease. There is at present no evidence of a deficiency of an NGF in Parkinson patients.

Another class of drugs called *neuroimmunophilins* offers hope to patients with Parkinson's disease. One of these, AMG-474, causes the cells in the substantia nigra to grow more connections to their targets. In animal models of Parkinson's disease, AMG-474 not only helps the symptoms but also retards the onset of fluctuations and dyskinesias. In the future, therefore, these types of drugs may be useful in delaying some of the complications of advanced Parkinson's disease.

NEW DRUGS

Although more than two dozen dopamine receptor agonists have been tried in parkinsonism thus far and all appear to be about equivalent, it is possible that better agonists may yet be found. The gene coding for the dopamine receptor has been identified; it is located on chromosome 11. It can now be cloned in the laboratory, and the intimate structure of the receptor protein can be studied in far greater detail than was previously possible. This will facilitate the search for new drugs designed to activate the receptor and could consequently lead to a new generation of dopamine receptor agonists.

TRANSPLANTATION

While experimental brain transplants will continue and improvements in technique will lead to better results, transplant surgery will remain experimental for the foreseeable future. It may become possible to take some of the patients' own cells and, by gene-splicing techniques, transfer to them the capacity to make l-dopa or perhaps even dopamine and then return them to the patient. These may be important therapeutic options in the future, but we should remember that transplantation of dopamine-producing cells at best represents a symptomatic treatment. The identification of gene defects in Parkinson's disease will put the question of transplantation in a new perspective. Researchers will focus on transplantation of genes or portions thereof by some means—with the prospect of correcting all defects of the disease, not merely the deficiency in dopamine-producing cells.

Appendix 1

Drug Finder

Tables 1 and 2 list the most commonly prescribed anti-Parkinson drugs, along with a brief description of dosages and formulations.

TABLE 1. *Commonly prescribed anti-Parkinson drugs (generic forms may have different shapes or may be available in capsules rather than tablets)*

Brand (trade) name	Generic name	Formulations
Anticholinergics		
Akineton	Biperiden	2-mg white tablet
Artane	Trihexyphenidyl	2- and 5-mg white tablets and 5-mg long-acting capsules
Cogentin	Benztropine	0.5- and 2-mg round white tablets and 1-mg long, elliptical white tablets
Kemadrin	Procyclidine	2- and 5-mg white tablets
Symmetrel	Amantadine	100-mg bright red capsule
Dopamine receptor agonists		
Dopergine[a]	Lisuride	0.2-mg, 0.5-mg, 1-mg white scored tablets
Parlodel	Bromocriptine	2.5-mg tablets and 5-mg capsules, caramel and white
Permax	Pergolide	0.05-mg ivory; 0.25-mg green, and 1-mg pink tablets; rectangular scored
Requip	Ropinirole	0.25-mg white, 0.5-mg yellow, 1.0-mg green, 2.0-mg pink
		4.0-mg brown, and 5.0-mg blue, all pentagon-shaped tablets
Mirapex	Pramipexole	0.125-mg white; 0.25-mg white scored; 0.5-mg white scored; 0.0-mg white scored; 1.5-mg white scored
Type B monamine oxidase (MAO) inhibitors		
Eldepryl	Selegiline (deprenyl)	5-mg white round scored tablets
Catechol-O-methyl transferase (COMT) inhibitors		
Tasmar	Tolcapone	100-mg tan lozenge: 200-mg tan lozenge
Comtan	Entacapone	200-mg tan lozenge

[a]Not available in the United States.

TABLE 2. *Levodopa preparations available in the United States and Canada*
(there are also many generic forms with different shapes, usually round)

Brand (trade) name	Generic name	Formulations
Levodopa alone		
Larodopa	Levodopa	Pink tablets[a]
		0.1 g (elliptical, scored)
		0.25 g (round)
		0.5 g (oblong, scored)
		Capsules
		0.1 g (pink and scarlet)
		0.25 g (pink and beige)
		0.5 g (pink)
Levodopa–decarboxylase		
inhibitor combinations		
Madopar	Benserazide/levodopa	Capsules
		25/100 mg (pink and blue)
		50/200 mg (caramel and blue)
		Dispersible tablets
		"625" 12.5/50 mg (pink tablets)
		"125" 25/100 mg (pink tablets)
Madopar HBS[b] 125	Benserazide/levodopa	Capsules
		25/100 mg (blue and black)
Sinemet	Carbidopa/levodopa	Elliptical tablets, scored
		10/100 mg (dark dapple blue)
		25/250 mg (light dapple blue)
		25/100 mg (yellow)
Sinemet CR[b]	Carbidopa/levodopa	50/200 mg (peach)
		25/100 mg (pink, not scored)

[a]Note: 0.1 g = 100 mg; 0.25 g = 250 mg; and 0.5 g = 500 mg.
[b]These preparations of Madopar and Sinemet are sustained-release (also called *controlled-release* or *slow-release*) formulations.

Most tablets and capsules have distinctive shapes, markings, coloring, and code numbers to facilitate identification. The letters and numbers are often very small, and a magnifying glass may be needed to read them. Some manufacturers impress the company name on their tablets and capsules. Others manufacturers print an initial or an identifying trademark or logo on their products. Generic substitutes may have a different shape or color. Tablets are often scored on the reverse side, so that they can easily be broken in half for smaller doses. The pattern of the scoring is often distinctive.

Despite all these distinguishing features, some pills may be difficult to identify. If there is any doubt about the identity of a forgotten bottle of pills, discard it or consult a pharmacist before using the drug.

Appendix 2

Organizations Concerned with Parkinson's Disease

NATIONAL INSTITUTES OF HEALTH

The National Institute of Neurological Disorders and Stroke (NINDS) in Bethesda, Maryland, plays an important role in Parkinson's disease. NINDS is one of the National Institutes of Health (NIH), the major U.S. government agency engaged in medical research and a part of the Department of Health and Human Services. The director of the NIH reports directly to the Surgeon General of the U.S. Public Health Service.

NINDS and other NIH institutes maintain a program of research in their own research laboratories and an active program of clinical research at the Clinical Center, a large hospital and clinic also located in Bethesda. A small number of patients are accepted there for special investigations and trials of new forms of treatment, including experimental drugs. Most important, NIH has trained many scientists who have gone on to become leaders in biomedical research in universities and research institutes throughout the world. It also sponsors a large-scale program of research grants to scientists at universities and research laboratories throughout the country. Some of these grants support research in Parkinson's disease and related conditions and basic research relevant to these disorders. For example, the NIH sponsored the *Deprenyl and Tocopherol Antioxidant Therapy of Parkinsonism* (DATATOP) study.

As we mentioned in Chapter 14, it was the fundamental biochemical work of Dr. Julius Axelrod and his colleagues at the NINDS in the 1950s that made possible the discovery of dopamine in the brain and its deficiency in Parkinson's disease. Dr. Axelrod won the Nobel Prize in Medicine for his achievements in this field. Most of the scientists who worked on brain dopamine in the 1960s studied with Dr. Axelrod. After his retirement, this work was continued by Dr. Irving Kopin and his colleagues, including Dr. Thomas Chase. In the 1970s, the NINDS established the Experimental Therapeutics Branch headed by Dr. Donald Calne, who with these fellows carried out many clinical drug trials and played a major role in the development of treatment with dopamine receptor agonists such as bromocriptine. Subsequently, Dr. Chase became Director of the Experimental Therapeutics Branch and carried out extensive studies on the metabolism and mechanism of action of levodopa in parkinsonism. The late Dr. Bruce Schoenberg, who directed the Neuroepidemiology Branch of NINDS, carried out important studies on the prevalence of Parkinson's disease in different regions of the world.

The NINDS makes available a summary of research in Parkinson's disease. A free informational booklet on Parkinson's disease is also available. Currently, this is NIH publication No. 94-139, entitled *Parkinson's Disease, Hope Through Research*. Copies and other news and information may be obtained by writing to the Brain Research and Information Network (BRAIN), NINDS, P.O. Box 13050, Silver Spring, MD 20811. One may call the office at (800) 352-9424 or find them on the Web at *http://www.ninds.nih.gov*.

NATIONAL VOLUNTARY ORGANIZATIONS

Voluntary agencies have been active for some years in sponsoring research in Parkinson's disease, providing information and educational materials, newsletters, and educational symposia for patients and their families. In the United States, there are several agencies operating at a national level, plus many large regional associations or foundations. There are also hundreds of local organizations, some affiliated with one of the national organizations and others operated by the patient-education divisions of local hospitals or functioning independently.

The major North American agencies are the following:

The American Parkinson Disease Association, Inc.
1250 Hylan Boulevard
Staten Island, NY 10305
Tel: (718) 981-8001, (800) 223-2732; fax: (718) 981-4300

West Coast regional office:
The American Parkinson Disease Association, Inc.
15000 Ventura Boulevard, #384
Sherman Oaks, CA 91403
Tel: (818) 906-7108

The Parkinson's Disease Foundation
William Black Medical Research Building
650-710 West 168th Street
New York, NY 10032
Tel: (212) 923-4700, (800) 457-6676; fax: (212) 923-4778

The National Parkinson Foundation, Inc.
1501 Ninth Avenue/Bob Hope Road
Miami, FL 33136
Tel: (305) 547-6666; Information lines: (800) 327-4545

(The Parkinson's Disease Foundation and the National Parkinson Foundations may have merged by the time of this publication.)
The Parkinson Foundation of Canada/National Office
Suite 316
4211 Yonge Street
Toronto, Ontario, Canada M2P 2A9

PATIENT SUPPORT GROUPS

Many regional and local foundations have been formed by patients and their families with the view of exchanging ideas and sharing advice on means of coping with practical problems. Some of these self-help or support groups have attained substantial size and prominence in their areas. Examples include the Dallas Area Parkinson Society; the Parkinson Association of the Rockies in Denver, Colorado; the California Parkinson Foundation; and the Parkinson Society of Greater Washington (PSGW) in Washington, DC.

The late Dr. Sidney Dorros, author of an excellent autobiographical account of his experience with parkinsonism, was one of the prime movers of the Parkinson Society of Greater Washington (PSGW). In 1981, the PSGW hosted a national convention of Parkinson support groups at which a national organization was initiated—The Parkinson Support Groups of America (PSGA). This organization was primarily interested in self-help and in developing grassroots support for the formation of a congressional committee on Parkinson's disease. The PSGA survives today in a number of local chapters, notably one in Montclair, New Jersey.

There are countless small local support groups in various stages of development. No fewer than 17 are presently functioning in the state of New Jersey alone! The American Parkinson Disease Association (APDA) and the National Parkinson Foundation (NPF) have information centers throughout the United States and Canada. The locations and telephone numbers of the local support groups can be obtained from the central offices of the larger organizations. They generally publish newsletters for their members, hold regular meetings, provide exercise sessions, and invite physicians, psychologists, nutritionists, and others to lecture on recent development relevant to parkinsonism. In this way, they provide valuable assistance to many patients and their families. The patient-education departments of community hospitals often provide some assistance and space for these local groups. Our own hospital sponsors several groups including one for caregivers and another for young parkinsonians. Some groups also raise funds to support research programs at various medical schools. They thus provide their members an opportunity to participate directly in the ultimate conquest of Parkinson's disease.

THE SOCIETY FOR PROGRESSIVE SUPRANUCLEAR PALSY

A small proportion of patients with parkinsonism, in fact, suffer from a distinct disorder known as *progressive supranuclear palsy* (PSP) or Steele–Richardson–Olszewski syndrome. Generally, patients with this disorder have participated in the activities of the various Parkinson's disease agencies. However, the Society for Progressive Supranuclear Palsy, Inc., was founded in 1989 by David Saks to focus specifically on the needs of PSP patients, family members, and caregivers. The Society is dedicated to stimulating research in PSP and informing members of recent findings. It publishes a quarterly newsletter, the "PSP Advocate," for patients and their families and makes available several information folders. A booklet, "Progressive Supranuclear Palsy: Some Answers" by Dr Lawrence Golbe is available in English and Spanish. Videotapes in VHS format are also available.

The society has cosponsored several international scientific conferences dealing with PSP, including a diagnostic workshop (held at the NIH) directed by Dr. Irene Litvan. Its executive office is presently at Woodholme Medical Building, 1838 Greene Tree Road, Suite 515, Baltimore, MD 21208. They can be reached as follows: Tel: 1-800-457-4777; Web site, *http://www.psp.org*; or via e-mail at spsp@erols.com.

Glossary[1]

Acetylcholine: Chemical messenger released by the cholinergic nerves, such as the vagus nerve.

Adrenaline (also known as **epinephrine**): Hormone secreted by the adrenal gland into the circulation in moments of crisis. It stimulates the heart to beat faster and work harder, increases the flow of blood to the muscles, causes an increased alertness of mind, and produces other changes to prepare the body to meet an emergency.

Agonist: See *dopamine receptor agonists.*

Amantadine: An anti-Parkinson medication; it may be used early in the disease or added to *levodopa;* has recently been found to be helpful in treating *dyskinesias.*

Angina pectoris: A characteristic pain in the chest felt as a squeezing or pressing behind the breastbone. It arises in the heart muscle usually during some activity and subsides with rest. It is a symptom of coronary arteriosclerosis or arteriosclerotic heart disease. The pain occurs when the heart muscle, as a result of impaired blood flow in the coronary arteries, fails to receive sufficient oxygen to carry on the work it is called on to do. Pains in muscles of the shoulder and chest are sometimes confused with angina pectoris.

Anticholinergic: Adjective applied to drugs opposing the action of acetylcholine. A class of anti-Parkinson medications that are mostly useful for *tremor.*

Antihistamine: Term applied to drugs opposing the actions of histamine and commonly used to treat allergic disorders such as hay fever and bronchial asthma.

Athetosis: Form of *dyskinesia* characterized by involuntary writhing movements, usually of the hands or feet. The movements are similar to but slower than those of *chorea.*

---

[1]Words italicized within definitions of terms have their own entries in this glossary.

Atypical parkinsonisms: Disorders related to Parkinson's disease in that they are characterized by *bradykinesia* and sometimes *rigidity, tremor,* and balance problems, but have other clinical features and other *pathology.*

Autonomic nervous system: A part of the nervous system responsible for control of bodily functions that are not consciously directed; for example, heart rate, blood pressure, sweating, intestinal movements, temperature control.

Basal ganglia: The interconnected cluster of nerve cells that coordinate normal movement, made up in part by the *substantia nigra, striatum, globus pallidus,* and *subthalamic nucleus.*

Benign essential tremor (ET): Condition characterized by tremor of the hands, head, voice, and sometimes other parts of the body. It often runs in families and is sometimes called "familial tremor" and "senile tremor" in the elderly. It is sometimes mistaken for Parkinson's disease, although there is no rigidity or *bradykinesia* .

Blepharospasm: Forced closure of the eyelids.

Bradykinesia: Descriptive term meaning "slowness of movement" (from the Greek, *brady,* meaning "slow," and *kinesis,* meaning "movement"); it is a cardinal sign of Parkinson's disease.

Bromocriptine: A *dopamine receptor agonist.*

Carbidopa: A drug, used with *levodopa,* to block the breakdown of *levodopa* to *dopamine* in the intestinal tract and in the blood.

Carepartner: Caregiver; spouse, child, sibling, or other family member or friend who participates in the care of and for a patient with Parkinson's disease.

Catechol-O-methyltransferase (COMT): An enzyme that breaks down *dopamine* at the *dopamine receptor* in the brain and that breaks down *levodopa* in the intestinal tract.

Catechol-O-methyltransferase (COMT) inhibitors: A new class of anti-Parkinson drugs that blocks the enzyme *COMT,* preventing the breakdown of *levodopa* in the intestinal tract by blocking intestinal *COMT,* thus allowing more *levodopa* to cross into the blood and then into the brain; examples are *tolcapone* and *entacapone.*

Choline: A naturally occurring substance that is a precursor of acetylcholine.

Chorea: Diagnostic term (from the Greek *choreia,* meaning "dance") applied to a nervous affliction marked by excessive motor activity ranging in severity from restlessness, fidgetiness, and twitching to flinging movements, sudden jerks, and spasms; it is sometimes associated with mental agitation. It is popularly known as St. Vitus' dance. —Involuntary movements, usually seen in Parkinson's disease from too much medication (see *dyskinesias*).

Cognitive function: The ability to think, to remember, to plan, and to organize information.

COMT: See *catechol-O-methyltransferase.*

Controlled-release levodopa: A formulation of levodopa that is released more slowly in the gut than the standard preparation, and thus lasts almost (but not quite) twice as long as the standard preparation does for any given patient.

Corpus striatum: Anatomic term (from the Latin, meaning "striate body") designating a large mass of gray matter deep in each cerebral hemisphere. Its internal structure and function are not yet well understood, but it is believed essentially to modulate or regulate motor and sensory activities of the brain.

Decarboxylase inhibitors: Drugs that inhibit or prevent the action of the enzyme dopa decarboxylase and thus hinder the conversion of dopa to dopamine. Carbidopa and benserazide (used individually in combination with levodopa) are decarboxylase inhibitors.

Deep brain stimulation: Electrical stimulation of cells in the *basal ganglia* that, instead of destroying, is used as a treatment for *tremor* (see *thalamic stimulation*) or other signs and symptoms of Parkinson's disease (see *pallidal stimulation* and *subthalamic stimulation*).

Delusions: Erroneous beliefs that cannot be altered by rational argument.

Dementia: A progressive decline in mental functions.

Diffuse Lewy body disease: Parkinson's disease that has spread to include many parts of the brain and usually is characterized by *parkinsonism, dementia,* and *hallucinations.*

Dopa: Chemical short name for 3,4-dihydroxyphenylalanine, an amino acid occurring in animals and plants. It exists in two forms, the L- and the D-forms (L being short for the Latin *laevo,* meaning "left," and D being short for *dextro,* meaning "right"). Only the L-form occurs in nature (see *levodopa*).

Dopa decarboxylase: Enzyme found in the nervous system and blood vessels that controls the metabolic conversion of dopa to dopamine.

Dopamine: Substance derived from dopa in certain nerve cells. It works in the nervous system as a chemical messenger transmitting impulses from one nerve cell to the next; it is deficient in Parkinson's disease.

Dopamine receptor: The area of the nerve cell in the *striatum* that receives the *dopamine* message from the *substantia nigra.*

Dopamine receptor agonists: Synthetic compounds that mimic the action of dopamine at the dopamine receptor in the *striatum*; examples are *bromocriptine, pergolide, pramipexole,* and *ropinirole.*

Dysautonomia: Abnormalities of the *autonomic nervous system,* which regulates such automatic functions as sweating, temperature, blood pressure, urination, bowel movements, and penile erection.

Dyskinesia: An abnormal involuntary movement, usually associated with excessively high levels of anti-Parkinson medication.

Dysphagia: Difficulty with or abnormality of swallowing.

Dystonia: Type of involuntary movement that is slow and twisting, and is associated with forceful muscle contractions or spasms. The painful end-of-dose foot cramp is a common example.

Encephalitis: Inflammation of the brain (from the Greek *encephalon,* meaning "brain," and the suffix *-itis,* meaning "inflammation," as in *tonsillitis, appendicitis,* etc.); it is usually caused by a virus infection.

Encephalitis lethargica: Type of encephalitis that occurred in scattered epidemics throughout the world from 1916 to 1926. It usually caused sleepiness, double vision, trouble swallowing, and drooling in the acute phase, and a special type of parkinsonism in its chronic phase. The disorder was also called *von Economo's encephalitis* and *epidemic encephalitis.*

End-of-dose failure: A loss of benefit from a dose of *levodopa,* typically at the end of a few hours.

Entacapone: A *catechol-O-methyltransferase (COMT) inhibitor.*

Enzyme: A protein or chemical tool that speeds up the rate of a biological reaction; *MAO-B* and *COMT* are enzymes that break down *dopamine.*

Etiology: The cause of a disease, or how it is acquired.

Festination: Walking in rapid, short, shuffling steps (from the Latin *festinare,* meaning "to hasten").

Freezing: Inability to move or getting "stuck," as with the feet appearing to beglued to the floor.

Gait: The manner in which a person walks.

Glaucoma: Disorder of the eye characterized by a sustained increase of pressure within the eyeball that can injure the optic nerve and cause impaired vision.

Globus pallidum: Anatomic structure of brain, a component of the corpus striatum. It is the target of an operation done to relieve some symptoms of Parkinson's disease.

Hallucinations: False perception of something that is not really there. In Parkinson's disease, they are usually things or people patients see (*visual hallucinations*), but occasionally, things they may hear (*auditory hallucinations*) or feel (*tactile hallucinations*).

High-dopa dyskinesias: Abnormal movements that occur when the *levodopa* in the blood is at its highest level.

Hypomimia: The masklike expression typical of Parkinson's disease.

Lateropulsion: Involuntary stepping or staggering to one side; it occurs in Parkinson's disease but can also be a symptom of inflammation of the inner ear.

Lecithin: Naturally occurring substance containing phosphatidylcholine; it may be taken by mouth to provide choline to the nervous system to increase the synthesis of the chemical messenger acetylcholine.

Levodopa: International generic name for the medicinal formulation of L-dopa (*laevo,* from the Latin, meaning "left") (see *Dopa*). It is currently the most effective substance available for the treatment of Parkinson's disease.

Lewy bodies: Round masses (about the size of a red blood cell) surrounded by a clear halo, or vacuole (open space), within affected nerve cells in the substantia nigra and other areas of the brain in patients with Parkinson's disease. They are a microscopic hallmark of the disease, identified in 1908 by Frederic H. Lewy, a German-born neurologist.

Livido reticularis: A purplish or bluish mottling of the skin seen usually around the knee and sometimes on the forearm in patients under treatment with the drug amantadine.

Low-dopa dyskinesias: Abnormal movements that occur when doses of *levodopa* are wearing off, or when the *levodopa* in the blood is at a low or falling level.

Mentation: Mental or *cognitive function.*

Micrographia: The small handwriting characteristic of many Parkinson's disease patients.

Monoamine oxidase-B (MAO-B): An enzyme that breaks down *dopamine* in the area of the *dopamine receptor.*

Monoamine oxidase inhibitor: (also known as MAO inhibitor): General term applied to a group of drugs that inhibit the enzyme that oxidizes dopamine, adrenaline, and related substances in the body. Drugs in this group enhance the effects of these chemical messengers and have mainly been used in the treatment of depression. —A class of anti-Parkinson drugs (e.g., *selegiline*) that blocks the enzyme *MAO-B,* preventing the breakdown of *dopamine* in the area of the *dopamine receptor.*

Motor fluctuations: The complications of the treatment of Parkinson's disease affecting ability to move; examples are *wearing off of dose, on–off phenomena,* and *dyskinesias.*

Multiple system atrophy: Medical term used to denote a group of disorders sometimes resembling Parkinson's disease. Various brain systems, though mainly the cerebellum, are affected.

Neurotransmitter: A chemical messenger; *dopamine* is a neurotransmitter.

Norepinephrine: A *neurotransmitter.*

Oculogyria: Spasm of the eye muscles causing the eyes to look upward (rarely downward) involuntarily; it is a characteristic symptom of postencephalitic parkinsonism following *encephalitis lethargica.* It has a sudden onset and may last for minutes to hours. Sometimes it occurs as a reaction to certain tranquilizing drugs, but it is never seen in Parkinson's disease.

Off: The state of reemergence of parkinsonian signs and symptoms when the medication's effect has waned.

On: Improvement in parkinsonian signs and symptoms when the medication is working optimally.

On–off effect: Descriptive term used to refer to marked, often rapid fluctuations from a state of parkinsonism to a state of normal movement and back again, which may occur several times a day. The effect takes its name from patients' comparing the experience to an electric switch being turned on or off.

Palilalia: Symptom of parkinsonism, especially the postencephalitic form, in which a word or syllable is repeated several to many times and the flow of speech is interrupted. —Stuttering or stammering speech in Parkinson's disease.

Pallidal stimulation: Electrical stimulation of cells in the *internal globus pallidus,* instead of destroying them, as a treatment for the symptoms of Parkinson's disease and *dyskinesias.*

Pallidotomy: Operation, done by *stereotactic surgery* in which a small region of the *globus pallidum* is destroyed to relieve tremor, rigidity, muscle spasms, and involuntary movements in Parkinson's disease.

Pallidum: See *Globus pallidum.*

Paradoxical kinesia: Sudden, usually brief episodes of marked remission of symptoms of parkinsonism that may last minutes, sometimes hours, and rarely several days.

Paralysis agitans: Formerly the official diagnostic term for Parkinson's disease of the World Health Organization's International Statistical Classification of Diseases. It is the Latin form of the older, popular term *shaking palsy,* which was used to describe the disease in James Parkinson's time.

Paranoia: An irrational belief that others are "out to get" an individual, making the patient suspicious and untrusting.

Paresthesia: (plural: paresthesias): Sensations, usually unpleasant, arising spontaneously in a limb or other part of the body and variously experienced as "pins and needles" or a feeling of warmth or coldness (thermal paresthesias).

Parkinson's disease: Form of parkinsonism originally described by James Parkinson: a chronic, slowly progressive disease of the nervous system characterized clinically by the combination of *tremor, rigidity, bradykinesia,* and stooped posture, and pathologically by loss of the pigmented nerve cells of the *substantia nigra* and the presence of *Lewy bodies* within the affected nerve cells.

Parkinsonian syndromes: Disorders related to Parkinson's disease in that they are characterized by *bradykinesia* and sometimes *rigidity, tremor,* and balance problems, but have other clinical features and other *pathology.* They are sometimes called "Parkinson plus" or "typical parkinsonisms."

Parkinsonism: Group of neurologic disorders characterized by *tremor, rigidity, bradykinesia,* stooped posture, and shuffling gait. The more common forms are Parkinson's disease and a reversible syndrome induced by major tranquilizing drugs.

Pathogenesis: The abnormal processes in the body that produce the signs and symptoms of a disease.

Pathology: The study of a disease process, including what is affected and what it looks like under a microscope.

Pergolide: A *dopamine receptor agonist.*

Phenothiazines: Class of drugs extensively employed in medical practice for various purposes. One group includes antihistaminic agents (e.g., Phenergan) and anti-Parkinson drugs (e.g., ethopropazine). Another, larger group comprises the major tranquilizers (e.g., chlorpromazine) that can induce a Parkinson-like state.

Pramipexole: A *dopamine receptor agonist.*

Progressive supranuclear palsy: Chronic disorder of the nervous system that often mimics Parkinson's disease. It was first described by Steele, Richardson, and Olszewski in 1964.

Propulsion: Disturbance of gait typical of parkinsonism in which the patient, while walking, steps faster and faster with progressively shorter steps, and then passes from a walking to a running pace and may fall forward.

Psychosis: A mental syndrome in which the patient loses contact with reality; psychotic manifestations include *delusions, hallucinations,* and *paranoia.*

Retropulsion: Involuntary stepping backward; the reverse of propulsion.

Rigidity (also called **plastic rigidity**): Descriptive term referring to the type of muscular stiffness encountered in Parkinson's disease patients. It is characterized by a constant, even resistance to passive manipulation of the limbs. It is due to a failure of reciprocal relaxation of the antagonist muscles. It may be felt as a stiffness by the patient.

Ropinirole: A *dopamine receptor agonist.*

Seborrhea: Increased discharge of sebum, the oily secretion of the sebaceous glands of the skin, particularly on the forehead and scalp, causing a flaky, red, itchy condition.

Seborrheic dermatitis: Inflammation of the skin sometimes associated with *seborrhea.*

Selegiline (Deprenyl): An anti-Parkinson medication, it inhibits one of the enzymes (*monoamine oxidase,* or *MAO-B*) that breaks down *dopamine*; it may be used alone as a first-line treatment or in addition to *levodopa.*

Serotonin: A *neurotransmitter.*

Shaking palsy: Older, popular term, used in James Parkinson's time, for the specific disorder now called Parkinson's disease or *paralysis agitans.*

Sialorrhea: Drooling.

Sleeping sickness: Popular term used during the 1920s and 1930s to refer to *encephalitis lethargica.* (Another commonly known disease, also called "sleeping sickness," is caused by a parasite transmitted to man and cattle by the bite of the tsetse fly. This disease is limited to Central Africa.)

Solanaceous alkaloids: Bitter-tasting alkaline substances extracted from plants of the family Solanaceae; among them are the botanical drugs atropine, scopolamine, and hyoscyamine.

Stereotactic surgery: Surgical technique for operating deep in the brain without opening the brain and without direct visualization of the site of operation. A long, needlelike instrument attached to a frame bolted temporarily to the skull is passed into the brain at angles that are calculated, based on anatomic landmarks, to bring it to a predetermined target. This technique makes it possible to produce very small lesions deep in the brain with considerable precision and minimal injury to the brain.

Striatum: Short for *corpus striatum.* Part of the *basal ganglia* circuit; it receives connections from the *substantia nigra* and contains the *dopamine receptors.*

Substantia nigra: Anatomic term (from the Latin, meaning "black substance") referring to a darkly pigmented area in the upper brainstem that can be seen on visual inspection of specimens of human and primate brains. Substantia nigra cells contain both pigment granules and large amounts of dopamine. —The part of the *brainstem* that produces *dopamine* and that degenerates in Parkinson's disease.

Subthalamic nucleus: A part of the *basal ganglia*; it is targeted by *subthalamic stimulation* to treat Parkinson's disease.

Subthalamic stimulation: Electrical stimulation of cells in the *subthalamic nucleus,* which, instead of destroying them, is used as a treatment for the symptoms of Parkinson's disease and *dyskinesias.*

Thalamic stimulation: Electrical stimulation of cells in the *thalamus,* which, instead of destroying them, is used to treat *tremor.*

Thalamotomy: Operation, done by *stereotactic surgery,* in which a small region of the thalamus is destroyed to relieve tremor and rigidity in parkinsonism and other conditions.

Thalamus: Anatomic term designating a mass of gray matter centrally placed deep, near the base of the brain. It serves as a major relay station for impulses traveling from the spinal cord and cerebellum to the cerebral cortex. —A part of the brain that receives information from the *basal ganglia.*

α-Tocopherol: Chemical name for vitamin E.

Tolcapone: A *catechol-O-methyltransferase (COMT) inhibitor.*

Tremor: Regular, rhythmic, to-and-fro, involuntary movement affecting a limb, the head, or the entire body that occurs at rest in Parkinson's disease. In Parkinson's disease, it may occur less commonly on holding up the hands (postural or sustention tremor) or when moving a limb (action tremor).

Tryptophan: One of the nine "essential" amino acids necessary for human nutrition; it is also the metabolic precursor of serotonin, an important chemical messenger in the *corpus striatum.*

Tyrosine: An amino acid occurring in nature and a normal component of the diet; it is a precursor in the synthesis of dopamine and adrenaline.

Vomiting center: Anatomic and physiologic term referring to an area of the medulla oblongata where several clusters of nerve cells initiate and coordinate the act of vomiting.

Von Economo's encephalitis: Another name for *encephalitis lethargica.* The Viennese neurologist, Constantin von Economo, is given credit for first recognizing and describing the disorder.

Wearing off: A loss of benefit from a dose of *levodopa,* typically at the end of a few hours.

Subject Index

Numerals followed by "f" indicate figures. Numerals followed by "t" indicate tables.